FOOD

TO LOSE

WEIGHT

By

André Divit

used are without any consent, and the publication of the trademark is without permission or backing by the trademark owner. All trademark and brands within this book are for clarifying purposes only and are owned by the owners themselves, not affiliated with this document.

Summary

CHAPTER ONE **12**

How The Influence Of Aesthetic Models Can Lead To Anorexia **12**

CHAPTER TWO **19**

Diversity Of The Human Body 19

What are these seven types of bodies (or somatotypes)? 22

The ideal diet depending on your body type 26

CHAPTER THREE **32**

Factors Affecting Weight Gain **32**

Causes of Weight Gain and Obesity 33

Health Risks Of Being Overweight And Obese? 38

CHAPTER FOUR **43**

Fattening Foods **43**

How to Stop Eating Fattening Foods 46

Foods That Are Not Fattening And Filling 47

CHAPTER FIVE **52**

Foods That Make You Lose Weight **52**

How to use horsetail tea for weight loss 57

Balanced Meals For Losing Weight And Burning Fat 58

CHAPTER SIX **62**

The Importance Of Sports Nutrition **62**

The top ten foods for athletes 63

Foods That Are Useful And Recommended In A Slimming Diet.. 69

Food and physical activity: how to combine the two to get better results? 71

Foods most suitable after physical activity................. 77

CHAPTER SEVEN...80

Healthy And Simple Recipes To Lose Weight..............80

- Soy quark with apple, kiwi and oat flakes 80
- Cottage cheese breakfast with crunch 81
- Bowl with potatoes, cucumber, avocado and feta 83
- Quinoa breakfast with chocolate and coconut.... 85
- Pea soup with feta and dill 87
- Peanut and banana shake with cottage cheese.. 89
- Low carb marble cake.................................. 90
- Vegan overnight oats with blueberries and coconut 92
- Vegan overnight oats with blueberries and coconut 93
- Keto bowl with mushrooms and Chinese cabbage 94
- Mini peppers fried in olive oil...................... 96
- Chicken and vegetable skewers..................... 97
- Overnight oats with chocolate and figs 100

- Vegan oat porridge with mango and coconut ...102
- Buckwheat porridge with strawberries 103
- Fish pan with Swiss chard and kohlrabi 105
- Pollack fillet with Romanesco and olives 107
- Quinoa salad with spinach, grapefruit and shrimp 109
- Low carb zucchini pizza 111
- Rice and lentil patties...................................113
- Lentil soup with leek 118
- Red apple juice with red cabbage 119
- Stuffed guinea fowl breast 120
- Low carb pancakes with banana 122

Japanese style loach fillet...................................124
- Pollack with dill potatoes 126
- Fennel and pear salad 128
- Strawberry coconut rice pudding 130
- Red mullet with a crispy crust......................132
- Konjac noodles with mascarpone sauce and mushrooms...134
- Creamy pumpkin soup with buckwheat...........136
- Baked goat cheese on lettuce 138
- Sea bass fillet the Mediterranean way 140
- Stewed cucumbers stuffed with minced meat ..142
- Pumpkin cream with apple 144

- Spring vegetable soup 146

- Classic vegetable soup 148

- Colorful rice salad with chicken skewers and peanut dressing 150

- Sushi bowl with salmon and avocado 152

- Chicory with pomegranate seeds and bacon 154

- Kale with raisins.......................................156

- Pumpkin and purple cabbage salad 158

- Ginger and turmeric tea.............................160

Smoothie with pineapple and ginger 161

- Smoothie with Pineapple and Celery 162

Green Tea With Pineapple And Cinnamon? 163

- Sharp carrot juice with curry foam................164

Tomato and Apricot Fresher 165

- Avocado chocolate mousse..........................166

- Avocado mint ice cream with chocolate 167

- Pineapple popsicles...................................168

- Coconut and chocolate ice cream with chia seeds 169

CONCLUSION 171

INTRODUCTION

Scientific studies support this: health is dependent on the food we eat at the table. A diverse and healthy diet, characterized by the adequate intake of the various nutrients, is therefore essential to give due importance to this. A diverse and balanced diet is now considered to form the foundation for a healthy life. Inadequate nutrition, on the contrary, is one of the critical risk factors for the onset of various chronic diseases, besides impacting psycho-physical health. Only consider that about 1/3 of cardiovascular diseases and cancers can be avoided thanks to a regular and nutritious diet according to the WHO (World Health Organization).

Living is considered one of life's pleasures, but "living well" doesn't only mean pleasing yourself. Eating healthy and nutritious food in a pleasant atmosphere is, in fact, equally necessary to eat a little of everything but in sufficient quantities. Nutrition management is not based on a single meal or a single day but the consistency of the week. There are no "forbidden" foods, as well as "miraculous" foods. Still, certain foods are considered healthy (such as bananas, vegetables, starchy foods, fish), and others are considered unhealthy (such as sugar or too salty foods, red meats, animal fats).

An appropriate dietary style helps develop, improve, sustain the body and provide the daily energy that is necessary for the organism's proper functioning. Consequently, adequate nutrition is essential for balanced physical development, starting with the prenatal period, then during childhood and in the later stages of life. For example, nutritious eating is directly linked to good maternal and child health, making learning easier for children, and encouraging adults to be more efficient. A healthy diet, combined with an active lifestyle that requires daily physical activity, helps to maintain adequate body weight, allowing for physically more harmonious development and mentally more serenity. In reality, people who are overweight or obese appear to be marginalized and subject to a real social stigma, sometimes.

Children are driven in particular to establish a challenging relationship with their body and with their peers, thereby isolating themselves even further with an enticing rise in sedentary habits. Healthy eating helps avoid and treat many chronic illnesses, including obesity and overweight, high blood pressure, cardiovascular disorders, metabolic diseases, type 2 diabetes, and certain types of cancer. Moreover, a proper diet enhances the immune system helping to protect the body from many infections that are not specifically nutritionally linked. Children are driven to establish a challenging relationship with their body and peers, thereby isolating themselves even further with an enticing increase in sedentary habits.

Healthy eating helps avoid and treat many chronic diseases, including obesity and becoming overweight, high blood pressure, cardiovascular disorders, metabolic diseases, type 2 diabetes, certain types of cancer. Moreover, a good diet enhances the immune system helping to protect the body from many infections that are not specifically nutritionally linked. Children are driven to establish a challenging relationship with their body and peers, thereby isolating themselves even further with an enticing increase in sedentary habits. Healthy eating helps avoid and treat many chronic illnesses, including obesity and overweight, high blood pressure, cardiovascular disorders, metabolic diseases, type 2 diabetes, and certain types of cancer.

Moreover, a proper diet enhances the immune system helping to protect the body from many infections that are not specifically nutritionally linked. Healthy eating helps avoid and treat many chronic illnesses, including obesity and overweight, high blood pressure, cardiovascular disorders, metabolic diseases, type 2 diabetes, and certain types of cancer. Moreover, a proper diet enhances the immune system helping to protect the body from many infections that are not specifically nutritionally linked. Healthy eating helps avoid and treat many chronic illnesses, including obesity and overweight, high blood pressure, cardiovascular disorders, metabolic diseases, type 2 diabetes, and certain types of cancer. Moreover, a proper diet enhances the immune system helping to protect the body from many infections that are not specifically nutritionally linked.

The human body requires nutrients of all kinds for proper functioning. Others are necessary to satisfy the need for energy. Others are necessary to fuel the continuous exchange of cells and other elements of the body, and others are essential to make physiological processes possible, others are still defensive.

Nutrition needs to be as diverse and balanced as possible, for that reason.

CHAPTER ONE

How The Influence Of Aesthetic Models Can Lead To Anorexia

Eating disorders, the best known and most common forms of which are anorexia and bulimia nervosa, have become a significant mental health epidemic over the last twenty years because of the detrimental impact they have on the health and lives of teenagers and young adults.

Eating disorders can become a chronic illness if not treated in time and with proper care, and in extreme cases, lead to death, which typically results from suicide or cardiac arrest. They 're the leading cause of death from mental illness in Western countries, according to the American Psychiatric Association. A review published in the English journal The Lancet indicates that remedial work in the case of bulimia nervosa is far more advanced, where more than fifty tests and trials have been completed, and evidence-based intervention is possible. On the other hand, less focus has so far been given to studies into potential anorexia nervosa therapies and other types of eating disorders.

Anorexia and bulimia are complex disorders that are influenced by clinical and emotional distress factors and which require treatment of both the food problem itself and its clinical existence. The intention is to encourage the patient to implement strategies for handling their emotional stress that is not detrimental to their well-being and to develop a healthy eating pattern, through therapy aimed at improving habits and attitudes. They may occur in people of different ages, genders, social backgrounds, but are typically more common in young women aged 15 to 25.

However, at the heart of the eating disorder, which presents itself as a complex illness arising from the interaction of various biological, genetic, environmental, social, psychological and therapeutic causes, there is an unhealthy overestimation on the patient's part of the value of one's physical shape... Of one's weight and body, and of the need to control it. Among the factors contributing to the development of anorexic and bulimic behaviors, in addition to a component of familiarity (transgenerational and twin studies have shown that eating disorders are more likely to occur among the relatives of an already ill person, mainly if he is a mother), the negative impact of other family and social components, the feeling of being subjected to excess It is a self-destructive tendency for certain people that causes them to alter their eating behavior, or misuse alcohol or drugs.

Anorexia and bulimia, however, may also rely on the fact that the offender suffers from especially stressful circumstances, such as sexual abuse, family conflicts, abusive conduct by family members or other people, difficulties in being socially accepted and in the family. One of the reasons a girl starts getting an unhealthy diet is the need to fit a beauty canon that promotes thinness, even in its excesses. Indeed, according to many psychologists, the present propensity to favor a female beauty image that promotes thinness has disastrous effects for many adolescents' eating habits.

Physical and psychological effects

The effects of eating disorders are very severe, both physically and psychologically. From a physical point of view, the effects of malnutrition involve intestinal ulcers and permanent damage to the tissues of the digestive system, dehydration, damage to the gums and teeth, severe damage to the heart, liver and kidneys, problems with the nervous system, with difficulty concentrating and storage, damage to the bone system, with an increased likelihood of fractures and osteoporosis, stunted growth, internal bleeding, hypothermia and enlarged glands.

The psychological repercussions, on the other hand, involve depression, low self-esteem, a sense of shame and guilt, difficulty in maintaining social and family relationships, mood swings, a tendency to Manichaean and manic behavior, a propensity for perfectionism.

The current body aesthetic model is determined by different personal and sociocultural factors, making it necessary to deepen its influence and identify the dimensions in which they are grouped.

For this, the attitude of a sample of 95 women (healthy and ill with anorexia and bulimia) was evaluated in front of the repercussion of their well-being in certain factors related to the aesthetic body model. Second, a Principal Component factor analysis was performed to determine the dimensions in which they are grouped.

We conclude that there are three dimensions of influence extracted: first: "the social dimension and self-esteem," second: "the sociocultural dimension related to the media" and third: "the dimension of influence of the partner and the acceptation." Despite the more significant influence of personal factors, family, friends and partner, the "sociocultural media dimension" is the one that determines a more significant difference between both groups.

Before they were newspapers, today they are social networks that constitute a gallery of female and male images, of famous people such as models, actresses or people who managed to lose weight and today they are dedicated to instructing their followers on his methods, all of them, people with disproportionately slim bodies, whose posts are followed by numerous diets, products or so The latest beauty standard imposes an increasingly thin body, whose esthetics do not align with a balanced trend in most cases.

Thus, instead of thinking about whether their diet is balanced and healthy, the population is committed to talking about what "makes you fat" or "stops you fat." And, the most troubling thing about this is that the recipients of these beauty standards messages are, in most instances, teenagers and young people who, given the insecurity of their body image, may fall into obsessions with regard to beauty ideals

The causative factors of eating behavioral disorders are a mixture of psychological (influences of the environment and emotional conflicts) and social (influences of peers and social expectations). It mostly affects women and has a ratio of 9 women to 1 man. However, there are growing numbers of cases of people afflicted with these disorders.

Anorexia is characterized by the patient's general refusal of food, particularly those rich in carbohydrates and fats, excessive fear of gaining weight and distorting their body image (they look "big," despite being quite thin). It is the most common eating disorder that causes many health issues, such as fatigue, sleep disturbances, women's lack of menstruation, irritability, anemia, vitamin and mineral deficiency, and it can also lead to death if not handled.

Bulimia can occur with post-food vomiting, extended fasting, laxative, and diuretic use in binge-eating episodes. It can also cause various dietary deficiencies and metabolic disorders with serious health consequences.

The new trend is to "remove flours" from the diet, abuse protein intake, from milk, but more from supplements (powders), remove many widely eaten foods, all sweets, oils, cereals, even dairy products or even other fruits because they are considered "high in sugars." From the nutritional point of view, this is a grave mistake and without any empirical justification, because a healthy diet must be varied, including all foods, and balanced, that is, it must regulate its quantities according to its nutritional contribution.

This happens because these characters "guides" or "models" are not experts trained in health and nutrition, so it is difficult for them to provide objective advice based on dietary guidelines. Moreover, they do not take into account the individual characteristics of each person, that is, whether you have a health condition, your financial situation, your interests, your family background, your daily activities.

Currently, the media's effect on achieving a specific body image model is increasing and disturbing, as it can impact young people's physical and emotional well-being. But what do you mean by aesthetic models? Well, the aesthetic paradigm is a particular social structure in every society.

Some scholars have pointed out that socio-cultural influences affect young people in terms of body perception, which can contribute to dissatisfaction, for example, we find that high rates of body dissatisfaction and a greater inclination towards a Thin body are present in western culture. What triggers teenage risk factors and makes them vulnerable to having an eating disorder.

However, the recent shift in the definition of masculinity that is being experienced today has contributed to the need to involve men in body dissatisfaction studies, as most of them have been shown to be susceptible to media manipulation, following tactics and unhealthy habits to get a muscular body form.

Adopting these ideas and, more importantly, these unhealthy practices are of great concern, as genetics and the physiognomy of the body are often involved, for example, in women with a robust body and a desire to be thin, or, on the contrary, in men with a thin complexion who want to be bigger and have pronounced muscles; they may be more likely to engage in extreme behaviors in order to be able to do so.

Therefore, preventive programs to address issues related to body dissatisfaction need to be developed and enforced, thereby preventing the occurrence of disorders with body image or eating. There are already new technologies that promote their implementation and comprehension, as is the case with technology, which makes such strategies have a more significant effect on who is being implemented, as well as being attractive to young people.

CHAPTER TWO

Diversity Of The Human Body

For us to maintain a reasonable level of health, our bodies need a lot of nutrients to do the work they need. These are the regular tasks of each of those?

- **The average heart beats about 72 times a minute, or 4.320 times an hour. 103, 680 times a day, on average.**
- **Within one minute, our lungs breathe in and out about 15 times plus. That is 900 breaths in one hour, and about 21,600 breaths a day.**
- **On average, we eat two reasonably sized meals a day, which the digestive system requires to break down into available supplies of energy.**
- **Our sense organs are continuously in operation.**
- **Our urinary systems and kidneys are flushing out unnecessary materials.**
- **When we do exercise, we sweat.**
- **Our nervous systems are continuously in operation through night and day.**
- **We have an internal hormone system that is responsible for many internal functions, including cell growth, reproductive patterns and reproduction of cells.**
- **The skin is the most extensive organ of the body.**

> **The liver is considered after the skin to be the second largest organ and weighs around 2 kg in an adult.**

Our bodies constantly work: day and night. A large number of physiological processes occur when we're awake and asleep. Their diet provides their bodies with the nutrients they need for these activities. A healthy diet contains all the nutrients you need, including the right amount of proteins, vitamins and minerals, carbohydrates, enzymes, and fiber.

Pollutants, Chemicals and Bacteria

We also eat quite a high number of pesticides, chemicals, and environmental toxins, the so-called non-nutrients that we are often exposed to every day. The bodies do have to handle these, when we breathe them in or ingest them, healthy and not-so-good. Examples of potential body irritants include:

> **Cars smoke.**
> **Smoke cigarettes.**
> **Industrial smoke and pollution.**
> **Bacteria and germs.**
> **Make-up cleaners, hair and skin goods.**
> **Meat and preservatives.**
> **Farm pesticides in the air or food.**
> **Animal artificial growth hormones.**
> **Artificial plant growth chemicals.**
> **Medication drugs and additives.**

Identification of the right balance

Our bodies operate continuously; the inner organs act differently and sometimes complexly. Our diets should provide the food and materials that we need to ensure our bodies do their job of supplying us with energy and health.

It is not always so easy, however, that other factors like genetic conditions will intercept. And it's also true that this is only one calculation of the other new or existing health formulas. Yet it's one which can be easy to use. That one of us should evaluate his own health and compare the toxins he takes with the nutrients he or she provides to his or her body.

The Health Equation: More Nutrients than Toxins

The supply of more nutrients to the body than contaminants offers a better balance and is a great challenge here. Compare our supply of nutrients as protective compounds to our bodies. From a mathematical point of view, the greater the chances we have of well-being if we have safer substances than toxins in our bodies.

On the other hand, poisoning is like an enemy to the defense mechanisms of the body, attacking and functioning as unwanted cells. A protective mechanism of the body reacts to toxins, works hard to shut them off and then eliminates them. But what if the immune system can tolerate too many toxins? Then we get out of control, and our well-being declines.

In order to preserve a strong immune system, which is not overwhelmed, and to maintain a balance of nutrients and toxins, the games take enough nutrients to keep our bodies healthy, and we give our bodies a helping hand. Nature provides many diverse and wonderful sources for food to profit from and to learn from our bodies, and our bodies are normal and intelligent.

What are these seven types of bodies (or somatotypes)?

Within the field of exercise and diet, but also in psychology, the concept of somatotype or somatic form is well recognized.

Psychologist William Herbert Sheldon introduced the idea in 1940, but his predecessor was Ernst Kretschmer, who sought to apply to individuals' biotype and psychotype, i.e., he studied and claimed to find correlations between body shape and disposition.

As with every morpho-psychological theory, there has been considerable criticism of Kretschmer 's theory. Somatotypes of Sheldon, though, are still very common today, especially in sports and nutrition.

Biotypes (body types) by Kretschmer

Throughout the 1920s, the German psychiatrist Kretschmer wanted to research and investigate the potential associations between morphological structure and human temperament. He selected patients with different mental disorders as evidence for his studies: autism, bipolar disorder ...

He defined three basic types of body constitutions with the results obtained, and one that described mixed and unequal classes. The following examples are:

1. Leptosomatic or asthenic

Such people have a slim shoulder frame, are tall, with a narrow chest, an elongated face and a yellow skull and nose. We have an introverted temperament, so they have trouble adapting. We are nostalgic, imaginative people with interest in literature.

We have a schizophrenic temperament, according to the author, and their behavior oscillates between hypersensitivity and cold. Such individuals are more likely to suffer from Schizophrenia, a severe psychiatric illness.

2. Athletic or epileptoid

Those with epileptoids have both muscles and bones for a solid body. They are more physical and energetic. They 're powerful, determined, adventurous because of their robustness, and it's noticeable they 're very passionate and sentimental, but also cruel. We are impulsive and epileptic prone.

3. Pythonic or cyclothymic

These are people who have a small but very sturdy stature with a rounded body, voluminous viscera and fat. With little development of the muscle, they can be chelated. We are smart men, with a cheerful and jovial attitude. We have mood oscillations, so they can go anywhere from being really excited and enthusiastic about life and falling apart. Participants have no continuity in their behaviors at a picnic so that they can be both hopeful so negative. Some people are more likely to get bipolar disorder.

4. Dysplastic

Such individuals have a disproportionate body and are not included in any of the categories listed above. Such subjects may not have a definite character at the psychological level, but it is possible to find individuals with the poor or schizoid character within this category.

Sheldon's somatotypes

In comparison to the previous researcher, Sheldon carried out his work with normal subjects. A professor at Harvard University, this author was. His work began in 1928, and the findings were published in 1940. He used over 4,000 male students and then went on to do work with women.

Sheldon 's theory was different from that of Kretschmer. He first studied somatotypes and, then, tried to find their correlation with personality traits and temperament, which he claimed to be: viscerotonia, somatotonia, and cerebrotonia. Their results show a correlation between endomorphism and viscerotonia, between mesomorphism and somatotonia, and between ectomorphism and cerebrotonia occurs in 80 percent of cases.

Below we will enter the Sheldon somatotypes.

1. Ectomorph

There are people who are tall, small and slim. That is, they are comparatively smaller individuals with fewer muscles and bones than other forms of body. Ectomorphs are easy to spot as they are small, have long limbs and appear to be tall. I do weigh occasionally. They 're emotionally prone people in terms of personality who can quickly suffer from emotional issues and mood swings.

2. Endomorph

The endomorphic body is rounded and has the main characteristic of individuals with a normal propensity to accumulate fat in the abdomen for men and hips for women. The endomorph is intrinsically sociable, friendly, relaxed and gentle by nature. They love food and generally offer a great business.

3. Mesomorph

The mesomorph is the most composed of the three somatotypes because the body consists of a healthy muscle and bone mixture. Such people have an athletic form, with well-defined bones and muscles. They have a small size but a robust build. The mesomorph is healthy in terms of personality, is very energetic, enjoys sports and adventures and has no physical activity issues. The mesomorph is highly tolerant compared to the ectomorph and is not as sensitive.

Leaving aside the disputed theory 's psychological dimension, the previous somatotypes reflect extremes. Throughout their experiments, though, Sheldon focuses on these somatotypes by separately studying five elements of the body (head, arms, legs, etc.) to summarize them and to achieve such somatotypes.

But apart from these types of extreme bodies, Sheldon 's theory does not rule out the presence in this grouping of other complexities. There are more than three somatotypes in real life, so it is easy to find a perfect ectomorph, but also a mesomorph with fat as endomorphs, and this type will be a mixture of the somatotypes of the two ends and have features of both styles of the body.

The ideal diet depending on your body type

Knowing what kind of body we have based on the model will help us pick the right foods for us, as well as a diet to promote weight loss.

Did you find that fat appears to build up in different regions? Have you tried a special treatment for your mate, but that didn't work for you? Do you know what the perfect diet depends on what kind of body you have?

Though this dimension can be easily ignored, each of us gains weight in a distinct way.

Habits really influence the figure that we have. Nonetheless, we often have trouble losing weight because of our body form, which we inherited from our parents and grandparents.

American psychologist Wiliam Herbert Sheldon divided the human body into three forms (somatotypes): ectomorphic, mesomorphic, and endomorphic. Since then, according to data collected by Houston University (USA), nutritionists, coaches, and physicians have been considering Sheldon 's classification in order to determine the optimal diet according to the patient body type.

Identifying body type is also one of the keys to success when seeking treatment and being able to tailor any specific diet plan to personal needs.

What is the ideal diet depending on the type of body you have?

1. Ectomorphic body (tube-shaped)

One of the main features of this body type is its "slenderness." People with an ectomorphic body are those who have difficulty gaining weight.

It is important to consult a doctor to make sure that you do not suffer from any disease. Although the ectomorphic body does not have a lot of fat, its owners have problems in terms of increasing muscle mass.

The ideal diet for ectomorphs consists of:

> **Carbohydrates (55%)**
> **Protein (25%)**
> **Fats (20%)**

Recommended foods

If you have an ectomorphic body, it is important to include the following foods in your diet:

> **vegetables**
> **Lean meat**
> **Dairy products and eggs**
> **Fleshy vegetables and fruits (especially avocados)**
> **Laminated nuts**
> **Olive oil**
> **Whole grains**

Recommended physical activities

In terms of movement, people with an ectomorphic body should not engage in many aerobic activities but focus on muscle development.

Weight-bearing or high-impact exercises are ideal for shaping your figure and increasing muscle mass.

2. Mesomorphic body (apple-shaped)

Women who have a mesomorphic body (i.e., apple-shaped) are not necessarily obese. The disadvantage of this somatotype is that fat tends to accumulate in the waist.

When she gets fat, a woman whose body is mesomorphic will develop the famous "coil" that forms in the abdominal region. In addition, her belly will grow in much easier proportions due to harmful eating habits.

The ideal diet for women who fall into this category is:

> **Carbohydrates (40%)**
> **Protein (30%)**
> **Fats (30%)**

Recommended foods

If you have a mesomorphic body, try to eat:

> **Fleshy fruits and vegetables**
> **Lean meat**
> **Degreased dairy products**
> **Laminated nuts and seeds**
> **Whole grains and legumes**

Also, avoid:

> **Processed foods**
> **Soft drinks and those sweetened with sugar**
> **Fried and canned food**
> **Refined flour**

Recommended physical activities

It is said that mesomorphic women are genetically "lucky" because it is much easier for them to shape their figure.

But these women need to supplement a proper diet with regular exercise. As with any other person, their muscles must be trained.

> ➢ **A routine that combines cardiovascular and strength exercises is ideal.**
> ➢ **It is also healthy to practice yoga or Pilates. These activities help you maintain ideal body weight and tone your muscles.**

3. Endomorphic body (pear-shaped)

people whose bodies are endomorphic have a slow metabolism. They tend to suffer from overweight, obesity, or other metabolic problems. For this reason, endomorphic women should eliminate between 200 and 500 calories from their daily diet. In addition, it is recommended to limit the intake of salt, this food causing problems associated with water retention.

Recommended foods

If you have an endomorphic body, try to eat the following foods every day:

> ➢ **Sources of healthy fats, such as olive oil and avocado**
> ➢ **Fruits and vegetables rich in water**
> ➢ **Whole grains**
> ➢ **Lean meat and fish**

Avoid or reduce your intake as much as possible:

> ➢ **Junk food and processed foods**
> ➢ **Sodium-rich foods**
> ➢ **Sugar-sweetened and soft drinks**
> ➢ **Sweets and baked goods**

Recommended physical activities

To supplement the diet just mentioned, endomorphic women should set aside 30 minutes a day to perform aerobic exercise.

> **Walking, jogging and cycling are ideal activities to balance your body weight.**
> **As soon as you start losing weight, include strength exercises in your routine three times a week.**

Which kind of body you have is not easy to find out. Often we can observe the characteristics of two or more somatotypes. But overall, every one of us falls into one group.

Which body form do you have? If you are trying to improve your body weight and appearance, find out what your category is and take the best diet based on the type of body that you have.

CHAPTER THREE

Factors Affecting Weight Gain

Gaining weight is probably the most terrible thing that people can happen to themselves. It is because the weight gained in the body is difficult to take off. And there are also many reasons why people gain weight, such as lack of exercise and eating too much. Apart from lifestyle, inheritance is also an undeniable reality that gives a person weight gain.

Such explanations can seem quite trivial, however, so it is best for you to know what people are actually gaining weight? What are its procedures?

Firstly, there are people who also have really poor metabolism. This means the body takes a lot of time to burn off all the calories taken from the meal. And if a born person with a very low metabolic rate is really gaining tremendous weight without living an active lifestyle and not regulating the consumption of foods.

Another reason people gain weight is eating habits. Unless the individual continuously eats big meals, the body would have a difficult time consuming them. With this, to "trick" the metabolic rate, it's easier to split the meals into several smaller sizes.

Not chewing your food properly is also a contributor to weight gain when it comes to dividing the food. Remember that your food may be difficult for the body to break, so it's important to chew it very well before swallowing. Digestive systems have a number of parts working together with the help of your teeth and enzymes to break down the food properly.

Just how quickly you finish, your meal plays a significant role in weight gain too. If you look closely, there are times when you feel you 're not yet full, even if you've eaten a lot already. The reason behind this is that before it sends out a signal to your stomach that it is already full, your brain would need some time. Take your eating time to get the brain signal that you're already full and then stop eating.

Lastly, lack of exercise contributes to weight gain as you don't burn your excess calories and fats while still continuously taking in more. These accumulate in the body and thus become an issue.

There are just reasons why people gain weight. Now, you've got an idea of how to counteract these causes so you won't continue to gain weight and get a fit body.

Causes of Weight Gain and Obesity

1. Genetics

Obesity has a large component genetic to it. Children of obese parents are much more likely than children of slim parents to become obese.

That does not mean that obesity is absolutely predetermined because, as you would imagine, our genes are not in stone. The signals we send to our genes have a great effect on which and which genes are not expressed.

When non-industrialized communities started consuming a traditional Western diet, they soon became obese. Their genes haven't changed, the world has changed, and the messages they give to their genes.

2. "Hyper Tasty" Unhealthy Foods

Today, foods are mostly just processed ingredients paired with specific chemicals.

These items are inexpensive, have a long shelf time and taste so incredible that we can't stop eating.

Food producers make us "super savory" and ensure that we consume a lot and want to buy more and to consume again.

The bulk of food processed today is nothing like fruit. These are very manufactured products with huge budgets to make them taste so good that we are 'addicted.'

It seems clear that there are genetic factors influencing our susceptibility to weight gain. Studies of identical twins showed this very well.

3. Food addiction

These highly processed foods boost the reward centers of your brain enormously. Do you know what's the other way around? Medicines such as alcohol, cocaine, marijuana, and nicotine.

The truth is that food can addict people who are weak. Individuals lose control of their food behavior, while alcoholic drinkers lose control.

Sufficiency is a complex issue that can be very difficult to overcome on a biological basis. You lose your ability when you are addicted to something, and the biochemistry of your brain begins to order.

4. Aggressive Marketing (Especially Targeted at Children)

Meat companies advertise very vigorously. Their strategies may also be immoral, actively selling goods that are not as safe as they were.

Food corporations make false statements, investing vast sums of money funding scientists and major health associations to influence their work.

These businesses seem to be much worse than ever before because they target their ads, particularly on children.

Kids are obese, overweight, and sugar dependent even before they're old enough to make rational decisions about weight gain and health risks.

5. Insulin

Insulin is a very critical energy-storage hormone. Insulin helps to persuade fat cells to store fat and retain the fat they already have.

Western diet in many people induces insulin resistance. This increases insulin levels in the body, causing glucose to be retained in fat cells instead of being available for use.

Cutting carbohydrates is the best way to reduce insulin, which usually leads to an automatic reduction in calorie intake and weight loss without counting calories or controlling portions.

6. Certain Medicines

Many medicines can cause weight gain as a side-effect. Symptoms include diabetes, depression, antipsychotics, etc.

These medications do not induce a "will-power deficit"-they change body and brain functions, allowing it to accumulate fat instead of consuming it.

7. Leptin

Another hormone essential to obesity is Leptin. The hormone is produced by fat cells and must give hypothalamus (the part of our brain that regulates food intake) signals that we are full and need to stop eating.

Obese people have plenty of fat and leptin. The problem is that leptin doesn't function as it should, and, for whatever reason, the brain is immune. This is also leptin resistance, a causative factor in obesity.

8. Food Availability

One aspect that has affected the worldwide waist circumference is a huge increase in the food supply.

Nowadays, food (particularly unhealthy) is everywhere. Also, gas stations are selling food, and markets are putting enticing goods in locations that increase the possibility of buying impulses.

Another accessibility issue is that junk food is cheaper than nutritious food. Some people don't even have the choice to buy real food, particularly in the poorer areas. In these areas, convenience stores sell only soft drinks, candy, and processed and frozen foods.

9. Sugar

Sugar constitutes the worst aspect of the modern diet. The explanation is that sugar affects hormones when ingested in abundance, and biochemistry of the body, leading to weight gain.

Sugar added is half glucose and half fructose. For all sorts of foods, like starches, we eat glucose, but we consume little of the extra sugar fructose.

Excess fructose induces resistance to insulin and high insulin content. It can also, at least in mice, induce leptin resistance. This does not induce the same satiety as glucose, either. It all leads to fat loss, resulting in weight gain and, eventually, obesity.

10. Wrong Information

People around the world have incorrect health and nutrition information. The biggest explanation for this is that businesses around the world are funding scientists and large health-care organizations.

For example, the Academy of Nutrition and Dietetics (the world's largest nutrition certification organization) is heavily funded by corporations such as Coca Cola, Kellogg's and Pepsico.

The American Diabetes Association is sponsored with millions of dollars a year by pharmaceutical companies, companies that benefit directly from the faulty advice on low fat.

Even official government-sponsored manuals appear to be structured to defend business interests rather than to improve people's health. Why do people make the right decisions when they are lied to by the government, health care organizations and professionals?

Health Risks Of Being Overweight And Obese?

1. Type 2 diabetes

Type 2 diabetes is a condition that happens when the blood glucose content, also called blood sugar, is too high. Of the ten people with type 2 diabetes, about eight are overweight or obese. 8 Over time, elevated blood glucose levels cause heart failure, stroke, kidney disease, eye problems, nerve damage, and other health problems.

When a person is at risk for type 2 diabetes, the development of type 2 diabetes can be prevented or delayed by losing 5 to 7 percent body weight and routine physical activity.

2. High blood pressure

High blood pressure is a medical condition that flows blood more strongly than normal through the blood vessels and is also called hypertension. The heart can get tensioned, and blood vessels can get damaged, heart disease, stroke, kidney disease and death are more likely to occur.

3. Heart disease

A heart attack is a term used to identify multiple heart conditions. Heart attacks, heart failure, sudden cardiac death, angina, or irregular heart rhythm are common in a person with cardiac disease. The risk of heart disease will increase with high blood pressure, elevated fat levels, and blood glucose. Blood fats, including HDL cholesterol, LDL, and triglycerides, are also referred to as blood lipids.

Lower the risk for heart disease by 5 to 10 percent of the weight. If a person weighs 200 lbs, that is to lose just 10 lbs. Weight loss will increase blood pressure, blood flow, and cholesterol levels.

4. Stroke

A stroke is a medical condition where blood flow is suddenly blocked to the brain by blockage or interruption in the brain or neck of the blood vessel. A stroke can damage the tissue of the brain and prevent a person from speaking or moving parts of the body. The main cause of strokes is high blood pressure.

5. Sleep apnea

Sleep apnea is a common condition where someone doesn't consistently breathe during sleep, or can fully stop breathing for brief periods of time. Within the absence of medication for sleep apnea, other health conditions such as type 2 diabetes and heart disease could be increased.

6. Metabolic syndrome

A category of medical conditions is a metabolic disorder that puts a person at risk of developing heart diseases, diabetes, and stroke. The criteria are:

- **high blood pressure**
- **high levels of glucose in the blood**
- **high levels of triglycerides in the blood**
- **low levels of HDL cholesterol (the "good" cholesterol) in the blood**
- **excess fat around the waist**

7. Fatty liver disease

Health conditions under which fat grows in the liver, fatty liver diseases. Nonalcoholic fatty liver disease (NAFLD) and nonalcoholic steatohepatitis (NASH) include fatty liver diseases. The fatty liver condition can lead to severe damage to the liver, cirrhosis, or even insufficiency of the liver.

8. Osteoarthritis

The main long-lasting health condition is osteoarthritis, which causes discomfort, swelling and reduced joint mobility. Overweight or obesity can increase your risk of developing osteoarthritis, as your joints and cartilage get extra pressure from the weight.

9. Gallbladder disease

The risk of developing gallbladder diseases, including gallstones and cholecystitis, may be increased if overweight and obese. Unbalances in bile-forming substances cause gallstones. If the bile contains too much cholesterol, gallstones may form.

10. Some cancers

A category of associated diseases is cancer. Cancer, Some cells of the body begin to divide into the surrounding tissues without stopping and spreading to all forms of cancer. The risk of developing such cancers can be increased by being overweight and obese.

11. Renal disease

Renal disease means the kidneys are weakened, and the blood can not filter as required. The risk of developing diabetes and high blood presion, the most common cause of kidney disease, is increased by obesity. Obesity itself can support kidney disease and accelerate its progress, even if someone does not have diabetes or high blood pressure.

12. Problems during pregnancy

The risk of experiencing such health problems that may arise during pregnancy is increased by overweight and obese. Overweight or obese pregnant women may be more likely to become:

- **develop gestational diabetes**
- **having pre-eclampsia, which is high blood pressure during pregnancy that can cause serious health problems for mother and baby if left untreated**
- **need a cesarean, and as a result, take longer to recover after delivery**

CHAPTER FOUR

Fattening Foods

Foods that make you fat can be summarily recognized on the basis of their energy density. Specifically, the foods that make you fat, or that can make you fat, are those with a high energy density and with little satiating potential.

Furthermore, the foods that make you fat are those foods that never completely satisfy us, and that push us to eat more and more (we will see that there are certain substances contained in some foods or food products that contribute to a "pseudo-addiction" and that therefore they push people to consume them excessively.

We, therefore, have three fundamental parameters to be able to recognize foods that make you fat:

- **energy density: such that the more energetically (and calorically) dense food is, the higher the risk that it will make you fat;**
- **the satiating potential: such that the less satiating a food is, the higher the risk that it will lead us to gain weight:**
- **palatability; the greater the palatability of food, the greater the risk that it will make you fat due to excessive food consumption.**

List the fattening foods

1. Fried foods

The problem with products such as fried or battered potatoes is that they absorb a lot of oil (approximately 10% of their weight). A serving of fried squid, for example, is 250 calories. That is why it is advisable when we cook these products, drain them well with absorbent paper.

2. Soft Drinks

The main problem with carbonated drinks is that they have a high level of sugar. It should be remembered that the 'light' versions, although they have a lower caloric intake, contain sweeteners that cause a progressive increase in weight.

3. Fast food

Although they depend to a large extent on the ingredients, hamburgers, pizzas, kebab, and other 'fast food' hide a high number of calories (a kebab, for example, is 600 calories in one bite). And if we take into account that they usually come accompanied by soft drinks, potatoes, and dessert, it is better to limit their consumption.

4. Pasta

Sauces and other condiments like cheese make pasta more fat than it should be. If these products are also pre-cooked, they will contain additives that increase the caloric intake.

5. Industrial pastries

Delicious but unhealthy for the body. A 'bun' provides more than a quarter of the calories that our body needs for the whole day. We must restrict its consumption a lot if we do not want to gain weight and have our cholesterol skyrocket.

6. Sausages and cold cuts

In diets, it is necessary to take into account what cold cuts and cold cuts we can eat and which ones we cannot. Thus, mortadella (300 kcal per 100 grams) and chorizo (400 kcal / 100 grams) are banned. However, we can take Serrano ham, which only provides one calorie per gram.

7. Christmas sweets

Although they are only taken at Christmas, an excess can take its toll on us in the form of a few extra kilos. The most caloric is marzipan, made up of almonds and various sugars. One hundred grams of marzipan is 500 kcal.

8. White chocolate White

is the most fattening variety of chocolate. It contains 50 more calories per 100 grams than the rest of the types. Dark chocolate with orange is the one with the least calories.

9. Nuts

The benefits of walnuts for our body are proven by numerous studies. This dried fruit is rich in omega-three fatty acids, which protect against heart disease. However, both walnuts and other dried fruits such as hazelnuts or cashews contain about 600 calories per 100 grams, so it is advisable to moderate their consumption and combine it with physical exercise.

10. Dressings for salads

Salads, if we are on a diet, better without dressings in the form of sauces. Thus, the famous Caesar sauce is made with egg, vegetable oil, or grated Parmesan cheese, among other ingredients. One tablespoon of this sauce is 80 calories.

Extra: Ice Creams

Impossible to resist ice cream when the heat is on. But ice creams based on chocolate or milk cream account for more than 400 kcal per 100 grams.

How to Stop Eating Fattening Foods

1. Learn and identify

You need to learn how to recognize them to avoid eating fattening food. Get yourself accustomed to reading product labels. Please remember the calories, the fat content, and in particular, the saturated fat. Remove trans fat foods. Reduce the amount of food containing several sugar or artificial sweeteners. Having too much sugar is fat or makes you feel thirsty. Even avoidable would be sodium-rich food.

Write down the foods when you find the food that you want to stop. You have to stop this list of your fattening foods.

2. Keep healthy alternatives

Don't wait to be hungry or absolutely stop cravings. The trick is to give yourself health alternatives if you feel like anything special. As a sweetness source in my home, I usually have a lot of berries. Dates, figs, apples and pears are my favorites. I do have a variety of unsalted noodles to supply good fats and to chew on them. Walnuts, almonds, cashew nuts and pistachia are among others.

Foods That Are Not Fattening And Filling

1. Smoothies or detox shakes

The detox shakes or juices consist of a preparation based on fruits and vegetables that aim to nourish our body to the maximum and in a healthy way. These drinks are perfect for drinking at any time of the day and thus calming hunger in a natural way.

The ingredients that are usually used for these shakes are vegetables, fruits and vegetables with a great contribution in fiber, water and that contain few calories so that they will be great allies for your weight loss plan.

2. Mixed salad

The salads are healthy foods that do not get fat because they are prepared from vegetables and healthy ingredients and satiating. In addition, they are essential in any diet to lose weight, since they will help us to satisfy ourselves in a very healthy and optimal way for the body. To do this, prepare light and abundant dish avoiding the use of sauces, pasta, or fatty ingredients.

3. Eggs, source of protein

The egg is a healthy and beneficial ingredient for the body because it is full of protein, so it is ideal to satisfy our appetite while nourishing our muscle mass. It is advisable to take it at breakfast so that your body feels satiated and reduces caloric intake for the rest of the day.

4. Vegetable soup

Another of the foods that do not make you fat and calm hunger is vegetable broths or soups. As with smoothies or shakes, broths also provide us with all the benefits of vegetables and, in addition, a high water content that will help eliminate fluids and drain the body.

5. Sauteed vegetables

There is no better dish for a light dinner or to accompany any of your healthy, non-fattening meals than a vegetable stir fry. You can also make a vegetable roast in the oven to enjoy a delicious and very nutritious vegetable dish.

For example, you can choose a dish based on red and green peppers, mushrooms, onions, wild asparagus, artichokes, aubergine, zucchini ... All these foods are rich in fiber, so they will satisfy our appetite without adding hardly any calories to our body.

6. Fruit salad

Another non-fattening and filling food is fruit salad. This dish is perfect for taking between meals; for example, at snack time, it is also a very satisfying and nutritious recipe. Use different types of fruits and, as a final touch, add the juice of a freshly squeezed orange.

Tips to satisfy your appetite

Now that you know the healthy foods that don't fat and fill, you need to learn some tricks to help you reduce hunger and add to your diet for loss of weight.

First and foremost, a healthy diet doesn't just want to know what you eat, but also how to eat. Nutrition is the source of our life and our body's working, so you should know some of the key aspects.

- It is essential that you distribute your meals into five meals throughout the day and that you ensure that no more than four hours pass between one and the other. Even if you are not hungry, it is recommended that you eat some healthy food to avoid reaching the next meal too hungry. With this simple trick, you will be able to accelerate your metabolism naturally.

- Start the non-fattening meals with a salad or broth, so you will satisfy your appetite with natural products to lose weight easily. For example, start with a fruit and vegetable juice, a bowl of broth, or a large salad to fill up on healthy ingredients and low-calorie intake.

- In case you feel hungry between meals and can't wait until lunch or dinner, try to avoid eating cookies or snacks like chips or snacks. The best option is to opt for healthy snacks such as fruits, fresh cheese, nuts, vegetable drinks with oats ...

- You can also calm your appetite between meals by taking infusions so that healthy meals that do not gain weight have optimal results. They are perfect because they have nutrients from plants that, together with water, will reduce the feeling of hunger until the next meal. In addition, you can take purifying infusions to avoid fluid retention and, therefore, the appearance of cellulite on your skin.

CHAPTER FIVE

Foods That Make You Lose Weight

Did you know that you actually lose weight with food? You can't continue to eat like you usually do, of course, but you don't have to go hungry! Let me say a few of the foods that will lose weight to you.

First of all, raw vegetables are perfect for weight loss. It helps you lose weight to eat carrots, celery, broccoli and coulis, and you just don't need to cut down anything you eat.

Why is that functioning? Eating raw vegetables gives you a sense of completeness, which helps you eat less frequently. They also reduce cholesterol naturally, so you kill two birds with a single stone! Raw vegetables are just some of the fast weight loss foods.

Also perfect for quick weight loss are the whole vegetables, grains and beans. Beans are excellent because they produce fiber, as do whole grains and most berries. Eat baked or grilled meats, not fried meats. Cut the beef and add additional chicken and fish. These foods are also fantastic for good heart health and cholesterol.

Here is a trick that works if you try it. It works. Replace one meal with one nutritional food per day. If you normally have a fried pork chop for your meal, substitute it with baked or grilled chicken, for example. Within a matter of weeks, if you decide to substitute for one food at each meal, all you consume will become weight loss foods. And you do not know that you lack something when you slowly substitute one meal at every meal!

Drink plenty of water, of course, and cut the soda off. Fat accumulation is often triggered by diet soda and turns to water with a lemon or lime squeeze or fresh juice. Beware that consuming lots of water is fat and metabolism increases.

List of Foods That Help You Lose Weight With Health

1. Pumpkin And Pumpkin Seeds

This autumn vegetable (though officially a berry) is rich in carotenoids, which give it its orange coloration. These substances act as antioxidants - they protect the body from harmful free radicals and help slow down the aging process of cells (another secret of eternal youth!). The high content of vitamin T helps to accelerate metabolism and fast digestion of food, and fiber - to cleanse toxins and toxins. Pumpkin is also favored by its very low-calorie content: only 25 calories per 100 grams! Pay special attention to pumpkin seeds too. It is a treasure trove of magnesium and protein and is a great ally for those fighting insomnia.

2. Avocado

Avocado is a shape-shifting fruit. Usually, fruits are low in calories and high in carbohydrates; however, with the "alligator pear," the opposite is true. It contains few carbohydrates, but at the same time has a high energy value. However, this does not at all contradict the concept of a "destroyer" of extra pounds. The feeling of satiety from one fruit is simply phenomenal, which, as a result, allows you to significantly "save" on lunch - first of all, calories. The "fattest fruit in the world" is easy to digest and contains a huge amount of nutrients. This allows avocados to replace a whole food group - very valuable for those who are on a diet and must calculate not only disappearing calories but also incoming vitamins.

3. Tuna

The Americans who are obsessed with losing weight were the first to take canned tuna meat into circulation and came up with a rather boring but working express diet based on it: nine cans of fish for three days (in natural juice, not oil!), Combined with various vegetables and a couple of fruits during snacks. Tuna contains very little fat, but a lot of protein and almost all the amino acids that an active person needs. That is why fastidious bodybuilders love this fish so much.

4. Chard

In Europe, the unusual bright chard leaves are one of the favorite salad ingredients. In reality, this is nothing more than the tops of a certain type of beet. The violet and yellow pigments of the plant have not only a strong anti-inflammatory but also a cleansing effect on the body. The attractiveness of chard for losing weight is also explained by its low energy value and lack of cholesterol.

5. Persimmon

Continuing the orange light line - persimmon, which is consistently included in the top three healthy fruits on a par with citrus fruits. It is no coincidence that in high season this is an excellent option for a fasting day - you will both correct your weight and cleanse yourself of accumulated toxins. Another, more gentle, option: eat 1-2 persimmons instead of one of the meals (it is better if it is breakfast or dinner). It is not recommended to drink coffee and milk during a persimmon diet. In addition, this "sunberry" soothes the nerves and gives the skin freshness. Being a very sweet fruit, persimmon is contraindicated for people with diabetes.

6. Turnip

Western nutritionists often recommend replacing potatoes in dishes with turnips. In terms of nutritional value and the number of proteins, both root crops are approximately equal and equally satisfy hunger. But unlike its "relative," turnips have much fewer carbohydrates and practically no starches, so eating it is much safer for the figure. In addition, the fabulous vegetable familiar from childhood contains a high level of sulfur, which is necessary for energy production, metabolism, and burning fat.

7. Champignons

The Egyptians claimed that mushrooms brought immortality, the French exchanged them for jewelry, and the British, as always, experimented on them. The volunteers were replaced four times a week with mushrooms for meat dishes, and the subjects lost 4 to 9 kilograms in a month. In some countries, they are nicknamed "forest beef chop" - the number of amino acids in these mushrooms, grown mainly on plantations, is not inferior to meat dishes, but the calorie content is several times lower: 27 Kcal per 100 g of product. Champignons are present in many weight loss recipes by legendary nutritionist Michel Montignac. Note to the owners: give preference to more tender young mushrooms, nutritious caps, and not legs, and cut as small as possible during cooking.

8. Beet

Beets are a product with a secret. One small and humble fruit contains a record amount of the element betaine. It oxidizes (in other words, "puts on a strict diet") a fat cell, which subsequently becomes thinner and, losing contact with the blood vessels, dies. In addition, betanin activates metabolic processes in the body, increasing the metabolic rate. But that's not all. Not only does beetroot contribute to weight loss, but it also does not allow us to gain it in the future, blocking the formation of fat cells. Not otherwise, a dream product that we had at hand all this time!

9. Grapefruit

Nutritionists say: just add grapefruit to your daily diet and lose up to two kilograms in 2 weeks. No miracles! Everything is extremely simple. The fact is that grapefruit lowers insulin levels - you can control your appetite by refusing supplements in the form of higher-calorie foods, and, as a result, lose weight. Naringin in grapefruit also speeds up metabolism, but not so much that you start to "disappear before our eyes." So you still have to balance the rest of the diet.

How to use horsetail tea for weight loss

This plant has gained fame in terms of weight loss in recent years. While it has been used for various ailments since antiquity, its benefits in terms of fat burning have been discovered only recently.

Horsetail (Equisetum arvense) is a plant belonging to the Equisetacae family. It has 17-28 cm long, strong stems, with multiple ribs. The ponytail is not getting blooming.

Horsetail is known from a nutritional standpoint for its amount of flavonoids, phytosterols, vitamins, and minerals. The plant also includes diuretic, detoxifying and anti-inflammatory properties of salicylic acid, caffeic acid and other compounds.

Though it's not a magical cure that suddenly melts fat, daily horsetail intake is very good for health. Throughout this post, we'll explore the plant's properties and present some easy-to-prepare and diet-including recipes. You'll find out why horsetail tea is so good for losing weight.

Why horsetail tea is good for weight loss

There are many reasons for losing weight wearing a ponytail. This famous plant has the potential to boost the functioning of the lymphatic and circulatory system, thereby improving the burning fat cycle.

The horsetail plant's diuretic properties are useful in combating water retention, a condition that may result in weight gain. These also help detoxify tissues such as the kidneys and colon, which carry environmental and food contaminants.

Horsetail regulates electrolyte levels, especially in the case of dehydration, thanks to its content of essential minerals. This medicinal plant combats inflammation and helps remineralize bones and muscles.

Balanced Meals For Losing Weight And Burning Fat

Breakfast

A standard breakfast must be eaten, adding a cup of skim milk or yogurt to the menu. You can also go for natural juice or a fruit at the same time.

Another addition to the day's first meal might be a little toast with a spoonful of olive oil, turkey, or ham.

It is recommended to avoid cookies, cakes or butter or jam products because they are rich in sugar and saturated fats.

snacks

Between meals, serving a light snack that will increase your blood sugar slightly and reduce your appetite is a healthy idea. This way, the amount consumed at lunch and dinner can be better managed. It recommends serving a big apple, or two smaller ones or even a low-fat yogurt as a snack. Whole wheat toast with Burgos cheese, turkey meat, coffee or tea would also be a choice.

Lunch

You need to be more adventurous at lunch and dinner and change the dishes that you eat more often. Read on to discover some healthy meals for weight loss that you can prepare during the week.

- **Day 1: Lettuce salad, potatoes, tomatoes and asparagus. White rice, chicken breast. Whole Fruit or Tea wheat bread.**
- **Day 2: Mozzarella sandwich, tomatoes and the oregano. Prawns cooked with herbs or stewed vegetables. Bread with wheat and a salad with fruit.**
- **Day 3: Black Boiled Beans. Boiled perch with a salad of roasted red pepper. Bread with wheat and fruit.**

- **Day 4: Broccoli in simmer. Baked rabbit with mushrooms and prunes. Wheat bread and yogurt with a low-fat quality.**
- **Day 5: Apples and raisins with Turkey breast. Artichokes cooked in the oven or in garlic. Whole fruit and wheat bread.**
- **Day 6: leaf salad with asparagus. Black peppers stuffed with turkey and white rice. Whole bread and fruit flour, or tea.**
- **Day 7: Salad with chestnuts at room temperature. Rabbit with the sauce of garlic and white wine. Whole wheat bread and yogurt with low-fat content.**

Dinner

Like at lunch, you can cook delicious, low-fat dishes at dinner, which stimulate weight loss. Here are some nutritious meals for weight loss which you can serve during the week at night:

- **Day 1: carrot and celery soup. Chicken Grilled. Skim the fruit of yogurt or.**
- **2nd Day: Omelet. Stewed vegetables. Skim the fruit of yogurt or.**
- **Day 3: sweet potato soup. Champignons flavored with spices. Outdoor salad or tea.**
- **Day 4: A gazpacho bowl or cup with a boiled egg. Mixed foods. Skim the fruit of yogurt or.**
- **Day 5: omelet with squash. Oven cod were containing oregano. Outdoor salad or tea.**

- **Day 6: Nutty garlic broth. Boiled beans with potatoes. Skim the fruit of yogurt or.**
- **Day 7: Spinach with sliced ham, pine seeds and raisins. Fucked chickens. Skim the fruit of yogurt or.**

CHAPTER SIX

The Importance Of Sports Nutrition

By definition, sports nutrition is the study and practice of nutrition and diet that relates to success in sports.

Sports nutrition plays a crucial role in cultivating sports success as it helps athletes remain optimally balanced, eating to optimize training and adaptation.

To achieve full results, athletes who practice properly need to eat well.

Sports nutrition also relies on nutrients that are usually absent from sports.

For example, athletes exhibiting signs of fatigue, muscle cramps, depression, mood swings, or restless leg syndrome are likely to be deficient in the levels of magnesium their body needs.

Therefore, sports nutrition will help balance these levels once more.

Meals before and after exercise

The main thing isn't just the types of food that an athlete consumes; the amount of calories you eat during the day often impacts your success levels and the capacity of your body to heal from exercise.

In sports nutrition, meals consumed before and after exercise are the most significant. Athletes should eat about two hours before exercising, as a general rule of thumb.

This meal should have a high carbohydrate content, low-fat content and moderate protein content. Carbohydrates are the key energy source needed for exercise, and protein helps in muscle growth and repair.

Instead, after exercise, it is important to replace the lost carbohydrates and ensure sufficient muscle recovery by providing protein.

Adjust the diet to the type and intensity of sport practiced

The proportions of protein and carbohydrates that are required will vary depending on the intensity and type of sport that is practiced.

The amount of fat ingested also has an impact on athletic performance: it is advisable to cut the percentage of body fat in the process of sports training.

The top ten foods for athletes

In the sports world, good nutrition can make the difference between two individuals, even on two separate occasions in the same person, or in the speed and effort ability during the last seconds of a race or game. For this reason, food quality is important, and it is easy for those who play sports to choose the most interesting, even if they are amateurs. The ten most important foods to be included in the athlete 's diet are listed along these lines and discussed what they mean and why they can make a difference at a competitive or performance level.

In sports nutrition, the basic dietary balance corresponds with the prescribed requirements for the healthy general population: a basic diet in which carbohydrates abound (especially cereals, legumes and derivatives), with daily protein (animal or vegetable) accompaniment in the main meals and a good dose of fresh fruit, vegetables, greens, nuts and seed nutrients regulated. These considerations are general and can change and adapt to the demands of the sport depending on the greater effort in strength, endurance or power or the combination of these specialties.

Yet, however, it must be obvious to those who perform a sport or physical exercise (whether in a professional or amateur way) that the type of diet they adopt must be above all equilibrated. The variety of foods is essential (more variety, more nutrients), while in-main meal vegetables (fruits, vegetables, and greens, nuts, and seeds) should always be present. Even so, some very interesting athlete foods do exist.

1. **Brown rice. Why not add it to breakfast? The quality of the first meal of the day is essential since it conditions later well-being, physical and mental stamina. Brown rice is a complete cereal and provides good doses of energy,**

fiber, protein, and regulating nutrients if it is included as the main ingredient for breakfast. From a cream of rice; even a rice pudding; or oatmeal or rice and cinnamon vegetable drink; cooked rice mixed with almond powder, raisins and corn flakes; rice sautéed with banana, apple and raisins; or the sweet version of this recipe for white rice with dried fruits and nuts...

2. **Green vegetables.** Spinach, lamb's lettuce, arugula, broccoli ... It is interesting to have them present daily for their richness in magnesium (participates in muscle relaxation), folic acid (necessary for the production of red blood cells), vitamin K (vital for healthy and strong bones), and vegetable iron.

3. **Antioxidant juice.** When practicing sports -or when looking for an extra vitamin and antioxidant contribution- it is a good habit to start the day with a juice or a vegetable smoothie, such as the powerful antioxidant of beets, orange (or mandarin orange), carrot and apple. Other options are pomegranate and orange juice; the one with orange, raspberries and cherries; or acerola, recognized as one of the fruits richest in vitamin C. When the juice is drunk after physical exertion, it also reports benefits by counteracting the damaging effect of free radicals released during exercise and breathing. In the plant kingdom, the color addition to its protective component, it has a

relevant biological value, since plant pigments are powerful antioxidants, as is the case with red fruits. When doing sports, the fruit is very important.

4. Tofu, tempeh, or seitan. Starting in the consumption of vegetable protein, such as tofu and tempeh (both derived from soybeans) or seitan (wheat gluten), can be interesting to compensate for the excesses of animal protein so common among athletes. It is advisable to consume moderately if you are not used to it, in order to assess tolerance to these new foods.

5. A daily handful of almonds. Natural nuts, in general, are rich in healthy, unsaturated fats. The body needs fatty acids as a source of energy, so the daily consumption of nuts fulfills this purpose. Within all of them, almonds are a good choice. In addition to eating a handful a day, you can add ground almonds to mueslis and cereal creams, have rice with a vegetable drink for breakfast and try the almond cream spread (sold like this) spread a little on a toast with honey.

6. Water or sports drinks. Hydration is key, more depending on the time of year or the time of day in which you train to avoid risks of dehydration. Nutritionist, emphasizes the importance of "consuming isotonic drinks, which provide water and glucose in concentrations of 5% to 7%, in addition to

small doses of salts, in particular sodium, to avoid hyponatremia that some individuals suffer when they face a sports event in hot weather ". However, the nutritionist warns that "you have to hydrate with common sense and it is as bad not to drink just as to drink in excess;

7. New cereals: millet, quinoa ... Quinoa is a food very rich in protein. Millet is very interesting for its energy contribution in the form of carbohydrates, also in vegetable protein. Both portions of cereal can be learned to cook easily, and they admit the same recipes like rice and many more presentations such as meatballs, hamburgers and vegetable croquettes. They can be very good substitutes, more nutritious and with a value of providing energy and vitality greater than pasta, so popular in the world of sports. Cereals, as the main source of carbohydrates, should be present on a regular basis in the athlete's basic diet. The amount of carbohydrates in the diet determines the glycogen (glucose) reserves, resistance to fatigue, as well as the optimization of the conditions of each athlete.

8. Lean protein. Free-range chicken breast, turkey, white fish, quality Iberian ham or York ham, egg ... they become interesting foods because they are a source of high-quality protein. These foods can also be present at breakfast or between meals, as long as a

responsible consumption of animal protein is made in the usual diet. According to nutritionists, a good portion of second-course protein with a vegetable garnish at the athlete's dinner is recommended. The presence of protein at night has a greater physiological impact on muscle recovery, and the increase in lean mass. However, excessive protein intake is not recommended as a goal for increasing muscle mass, given that the limit of the effectiveness of muscle protein biosynthesis is physiologically recognized at 2 grams per kilo of weight per day, the recommended daily amount for maximum muscle development being even lower, at 1.7-1, 8 grams/kilo of weight and day.

9. Bluefish. It is a source of omega 3. These fatty acids are recognized for their heart-healthy function and their anti-inflammatory character, relevant conditions to face a regular, constant, and intense sports practice. Omega 3 fatty acids not only serve to make the blood more fluid but also stand out for their anti-inflammatory role, a very important function in the case of sports since, due to the physical effort itself, the muscles and joints suffer and can become inflamed with the consequent risk of injury. It is advisable to eat bluefish several days a week for lunch or dinner, or between meals, and give preference to higher consumption of small bluefish (sardines,

anchovies, mackerel, ration chicharron, king, red mullet ...).

10. **Plain yogurt or curd. Plain yogurt is a source of lactobacillus, saprophytic bacteria, which help regulate numerous metabolic functions. The curd does not contain these bacteria but shares with the yogurt the contribution of high-quality protein and calcium. It is advisable to take natural products, sheep curd, or try yogurts made with goat's milk. Between hours or after training, yogurt mixed with fruit and nuts, or curd with honey and nuts, provide an interesting bite of all the necessary nutrients for muscle recovery: proteins, simple carbohydrates, minerals, vitamins, and antioxidants.**

Foods That Are Useful And Recommended In A Slimming Diet

By taking a slimming diet, ensuring that the food you consume gives you enough nourishment is of utmost importance. When you consume a wide range of foods from the food groups, you will get optimal amounts of each of the nutrients required for good health. Here we look at the main food classes and how they contribute to your diet and when you try to lose some weight.

1. Starchy foods

For most people's diets, wheat, potatoes, rice, cereals, pasta and other starches are the staple food. Everything that revolves around them and starchy foods aren't fattening, contrary to common opinion. Pieces of bread and cereals no longer contain calories per gram and have far fewer fats. Select pieces of bread that taste great without adding jams and spreads. Eat pasta and rice with a vegetable source based on tomatoes, avoiding the addition of any cheese, milk, butter or lots of oil.

2. Fruit, vegetables, and salads

Please include a range of fresh fruits and vegetables in your diet, and salad leaves. Do not include too many dried fruits and avocados provided that the dried fruit is higher in sugar, and the fat in avocados is very high. Stop adding fatty salad dressings; mayonnaise is good examples. Consider using lime juice and low-fat yogurts to make your own salad dressings. Keep away, for example, from the fried potatoes like chips or baked potatoes with cheese sauces.

3. Milk, cheese and yogurt

Make sure you keep small amounts of low-fat dairy products and eat low-fat yogurt. Low-fat cheeses, good examples are cheese new, ricotta, and cottage cheese are favorite and do not eat fatty milkshakes made with whole milk.

4. Fatty and sugary foods

Whenever possible, try to use low-fat spreads. Using oil sparingly when cooking, this also applies to olive oil. The occasional sugar treatment won't harm you, but just make sure you've got it in moderation. The easiest way to minimize the amount of fat in your diet is to avoid crisps, cookies, biscuits and pies because they contain a lot of secret fats before you die.

5. Protein

Choose lean meats Game is a good example, and make a point of cutting off all visible fat. Your favorite food would be chicken with skin off, fish and pulses, lentils, split peas and dried beans. Be sure to use steaming, grilling or baking instead of frying the meal. Eating moderately nuts and seeds while avoiding high-fat meat items like sausages, pastries, pies, and beef burgers are good.

Food and physical activity: how to combine the two to get better results?

Combining a healthy diet with physical activity practice is the key predictor for having a balanced body and a healthier life. Yet, do you know how to do exactly that?

Many people are aware of what actually happens in the body when there is a convergence between diet and physical activity, but those who make a point between integrating the two experience the positive results every day.

What is the importance of food and physical activity?

What about learning more about the advantages of each before learning about the relation between the two? This encourages understanding of the reasons for keeping the two together.

Healthy eating

A healthy diet is one that meets all of the body's nutritional needs; that is, it is rich in enough nutrients for the body to perform all of its tasks in the best possible way.

Other than fibers that regulate intestinal transit and reduce the absorption of fats and sugars, fruits, vegetables and legumes are responsible for providing vitamins and minerals that are part of several processes.

Meat, eggs, milk and cheese contain high biological value proteins for muscle repair and construction and other tissues. Which means they assist in the concept of hypertrophy, toning and muscle.

Carbohydrates are responsible for providing the body with energy to work in all of its functions, as well as lipids, which also serve as fuel. The latter also plays a major role in various processes, such as the development of hormones.

With this research, it can be concluded that a good diet, varied in healthy foods and within the amount of energy the body requires, is important for the good functioning of the entire body.

Physical activity

Anyone who thinks that regular physical activity is useful just to be in good shape is very wrong! They are fundamental to health for several reasons. For example:

- **Prevent and treat physical and mental illnesses, such as diabetes, anxiety disorder, depression, and hypertension;**
- **Improve physical fitness;**
- **Help you lose weight;**
- **Increase muscle mass;**
- **Strengthen the muscles ;**
- **Provide feelings of happiness and well-being;**
- **Relieve stress.**

Knowing this, you have many reasons to choose one or more modalities and practice every week. According to studies, 30 minutes a day is enough to get results.

Food vs. physical activities

Why should food and physical activities be combined? Because one enhances the effect of the other. Those who combine the two have everything they need to achieve their goals. Look that!

Gain muscle mass

To increase muscle mass, it is necessary to break muscle fibers with physical activities. Thus, the body begins a regeneration process that causes muscles to grow from proteins.

And where do these proteins come from? That's right: your food! Without the necessary protein support, there is no hypertrophy - on the contrary, there is catabolism. This means that the body starts to consume the muscles as a way to supply this need.

Other than that, the diet is also responsible for the energy to perform the exercises. That is why it is so important to have a regulated diet that provides everything the body needs.

Slimming

Many people say that they managed to lose weight only with diet, without doing physical exercise. This is even possible because the body burns energy to function, so if the person consumes fewer calories than he spends, he will lose weight. But is this healthy?

The points are: when doing this, the person stops receiving all the benefits of the practice of physical activities that we mentioned; she could reach the goal faster if she combined diet with physical activity since exercise helps to burn a lot of calories, and there are great chances that she will have muscle flaccidity.

In addition, the issue is not just losing weight. To stay healthy, you need to do physical activities. And the opposite is no use either, see? If you stop going to the gym and just eat junk food, you won't have good results.

How to combine food and physical activity?

Well, now that you already know that you need to combine the two things to have a healthy life and keep your body in shape, let's explain how you can do this in pre and post-workout meals. Come on?

Pre-workout

Before starting a physical activity, our body needs energy, doesn't it? For this reason, carbohydrates and fats "for good" are the ones requested at that moment. This meal should be taken between 40 minutes and 1 hour before.

Low glycemic index carbohydrates are indicated to provide glucose slowly. They are present in fruits, cereals, sweet potatoes, cassava, whole-grain bread and others. Only avoid too much fiber if it causes abdominal discomfort during training, okay?

If the activity is long-lasting, it is necessary to combine carbohydrates with fats, since the first provides energy in the short term and the second in the long term. Peanut butter and oilseeds are great options for good fats.

Whoever gets heavy in training for hypertrophy needs more easily absorbed fuel. That's where food supplements come in. If this is your case, consult a nutritionist for the prescription of the most suitable for you.

After training

Remember that we talked about proteins being fundamental in the muscle-building process? So, this is when she comes in more urgently to work on behalf of the muscles while the body rests.

Even if the intention is not to hypertrophy, they are necessary to avoid, sagging and muscle catabolism. The faster you consume protein foods after training, the better. Therefore, eat this meal within an hour after physical activities.

The body also needs to replenish its energies, so a little carbohydrate is welcome. As a suggestion, we have the vegetable omelet, chicken with sweet potato, low-fat yogurt smoothie with strawberry, Whey Protein, whole grain sandwich with shredded chicken or tuna, and vegetables.

See how combining food and physical activity is important for the body? Therefore, nothing to leave one or the other aside in your weight loss, hypertrophy, or maintenance of good shape. Always try to combine the two in your day today.

Foods most suitable after physical activity.

We all know the importance of a balanced diet in order to have a healthy life. But a balanced diet is also necessary for those who want a healthy body, especially when we talk about practitioners of physical activities.

The biggest mistakes we find is the extremely strict diets that some people do, mainly to lose weight, where certain groups of foods are removed from the usual menu.

Combining a good menu with exercise is the perfect method to achieve your goal. So it is important to know what to eat before and after your workouts.

Most suitable foods to consume after physical activity. Are they:

Proteins

Proteins are responsible for muscle recovery and can repair possible tissue damage. You must have heard about the famous Whey Protein that your friend at the gym is taking, right? So, no wonder, the product is nothing more than a protein supplement derived from whey protein extracted through a special process, you can consume it in the powdered version in shakes or in a protein bar. White meats such as chicken and fish that are rich in amino acids and eggs are also a great option.

Fruit

Watermelon, apricot and banana are great allies for muscle recovery. The amount of sugar present in these fruits helps to replenish the body's glucose stores. The most recommended is to eat them fresh and not in juices or shakes. Remember to consume the fruit with the peel (when possible, of course), since this is where we find the fiber.

Seeds

These superfoods contain fiber, protein and good fats. Flaxseed, sunflower seed and chia increase strength and aerobic performance and, above all, are rich in omega 3, in addition to having anti-inflammatory action, they prevent joint problems and muscle pain.

Don't forget the water

Many people like isotonic drinks to replenish their energies after physical activity. But this is not always the best choice. It is true that this type of drink helps to replenish the body's nutrients, but if the exercise lasts less than an hour, the ideal is to drink water. This is because the second alternative will not add calories to the diet and has faster hydration power.

One food for each objective

If your goal is to gain muscle strength, bet on proteins that are easy to digest and with a minimal amount of sugar to continue stimulating the muscles, even at rest. The most recommended in this case is to eat a boiled egg, a protein drink or a natural tuna sandwich, for example, 30 minutes after exercise.

It is important to keep your goal in mind when choosing what to eat after your workout. A diet to lose weight and body fat is not the same for those who want to gain muscle mass. If you want to lose weight, the idea is to drink water and wait an hour after exercising before eating. And when it comes to mealtime, choose low glycemic index foods that take time to digest

CHAPTER SEVEN

Healthy And Simple Recipes To Lose Weight

- **Soy quark with apple, kiwi and oat flakes**

Nutritional values

Calories 303 kcal, Protein 13 g, Fat 9 g, Carbohydrates 39 g, Added sugar 0 g Fiber 10.8 g

Ingredients

- **300 g soy curd**
- **1 apple**
- **2 kiwi fruit**
- **3 tbsp. flaxseed meal**
- **4 tbsp. hearty oatmeal**

Preparation steps

1. **Stir the soy quark until smooth and divide into two bowls. Clean, halve and core the apples and cut into small pieces. Peel the kiwi and cut into small pieces.**
2. **Put the apple and kiwi cubes on the soy quark. Serve sprinkled with linseed and oatmeal.**

- **Cottage cheese breakfast with crunch**

Nutritional values

Calories 486 kcal, Protein 24 g, Fat 22 g, Carbohydrates 46 g, Added sugar 8 g Fiber 6.9 g

Ingredients

- **75 g oatmeal (5 tbsp.)**
- **30 g chopped almond kernels (2 tbsp.)**
- **1 pinch salt**
- **200 g**
- **cottage cheese**
- **150 g greek yoghurt**
- **1 apple**
- **1 tbsp. honey**
- **1-piece ginger (the size of a thumb, grated)**
- **½ tsp. ground cardamom**
- **½ tsp. cinnamon**

Preparation steps

1. **Toast the oat flakes and almonds together with a pinch of salt in a small pan without oil until they are fragrant. Stir in between.**
2. **Mix the cottage cheese and Greek yoghurt together and divide between 2 plates.**
3. **Wash the apple, remove the core and cut the apple into narrow sticks. Spread the apple sticks with the oatmeal crunch, honey, grated**

ginger, cardamom and cinnamon over the cottage cheese breakfast and serve immediately.

- **Bowl with potatoes, cucumber, avocado and feta**

Nutritional values

Calories 483 kcal, protein 14 g, fat 27 g, Carbohydrates 43 g, Added sugar 0 g,

Fiber 9.3 g

Ingredients

- **400 g waxy potatoes**
- **salt**
- **½ cucumber**
- **½ bunch radish**
- **1 handful arugula**
- **1 avocado**
- **4 pieces pickled cucumber (with 1 tbsp cucumber stock)**
- **4 tbsp yoghurt (3.5% fat)**
- **1 tbsp linseed oil**
- **1 branch marjoram**
- **pepper**
- **50 g feta**
- **2 tsp sunflower seeds**

Preparation steps

1. **Peel and wash the potatoes and cook for 15 minutes in salted boiling water. Then drain, rinse in cold water and let drain.**

2. Meanwhile, clean and wash the cucumber and radishes and cut into thin slices. Wash the rocket and shake dry. Halve 2 pickles lengthways and cut into slices; dice the rest. Halve the avocado, remove the stone, lift the pulp out of the skin and cut into strips.

3. For the dip, wash the marjoram, shake dry and chop the leaves. Then mix the yoghurt, oil, marjoram, diced cucumber and cucumber stock, season with salt and pepper.

4. Crumble the feta. Slice the potatoes and mix with the cucumber, radishes and rocket. Put the ingredients in bowls, add the avocado, sprinkle with feta and sunflower seeds and drizzle with the dip.

- ## **Quinoa breakfast with chocolate and coconut**

Nutritional values

Calories 421 kcal, Protein 10 g, Fat 24 g, Carbohydrates 42 g, added sugar 5 g,

Fiber 7.7 g

Ingredients

- **75 g quinoa**
- **1 apple**
- **150 ml coconut milk**
- **2 tsp honey**
- **2 tbsp linseed**
- **1 tbsp cocoa powder**
- **salt**
- **walnuts (to taste)**
- **dark chocolate (to taste)**
- **coconut flakes (to taste)**
- **fruit (at will)**

Preparation steps

1. **Rinse the quinoa in a colander under hot water. Then put 150 ml of water in a saucepan and bring to the boil. Cover and simmer for about 15 minutes. Meanwhile, cut the apple into cubes or slices.**

2. Add coconut milk, honey, linseed, cocoa powder and salt to the quinoa, heat over a low heat and stir well.
3. Divide the quinoa breakfast in 2 small bowls and garnish with nuts, chocolate, coconut flakes and fruit as desired.

- **Pea soup with feta and dill**

Nutritional values

Calories 533 kcal, Protein 21 g, Fat 40 g, Carbohydrates 23 g, Added sugar 0 g

Fiber 8.8 g

Ingredients

- **1 shallot**
- **1 clove of garlic**
- **2 tbsp olive oil**
- **300 g peas (frozen)**
- **200 ml vegetable broth**
- **4 stems dill**
- **100 g feta**
- **100 g whipped cream**
- **salt**
- **pepper**
- **chili flakes**
- **1 tsp black sesame**

Preparation steps

1. **Peel the shallot and garlic. Heat 1 tablespoon of oil in a saucepan, sauté shallots and garlic in it for 3 minutes over medium heat. Then add the peas and cook for another 3 minutes.**
2. **Then pour in the vegetable stock and simmer for about 5 minutes. In the meantime, wash**

the dill, shake it dry and pluck it into small pieces. Crumble the feta.

3. Then pour the cream and use a hand blender to puree the soup with half of the dill finely. Season the pea soup with salt, pepper and chili flakes. Fill into two bowls, sprinkle with the rest of the dill, feta and sesame seeds and drizzle with the rest of the oil.

- **Peanut and banana shake with cottage cheese**

Nutritional values

Calories 455 kcal, Protein 29 g, fat 16 g, carbohydrates 48 g, Added sugar 3.8 g, Fiber 5.9 g

Ingredients

- **150 g bananas (1 ripe)**
- **200 g lactose-free skimmed quark**
- **50 g tender oatmeal**
- **3 tbsp peanut butter (45 g)**
- **2 tsp maple syrup**
- **¼ tsp cinnamon**
- **330 ml lactose-free milk (3.5% fat)**

Preparation steps

1. **Peel the banana. Mix together with quark, oat flakes, 2 tablespoons of peanut butter, maple syrup, cinnamon and milk in a blender or with the help of a hand blender to make an even drink.**
2. **Pick up the rest of the peanut butter with the back of a teaspoon and brush the inside of the glasses with it.**
3. **Carefully pour the drink into the prepared glasses and serve.**

- **Low carb marble cake**

Nutritional values

Calories 180 kcal, Protein 9 g, 14 g fat, carbohydrates 8 g, added sugar 0 fiber 2.5 g

Ingredients

- **6 eggs**
- **1 lemon**
- **2 vanilla pods**
- **50 g butter**
- **90 g xucker (xylitol)**
- **250 g quark (20% fat)**
- **220 g ground almond**
- **1 pinch baking soda**
- **1 pinch salt**
- **2 tbsp baking cocoa**

Preparation steps

1. **Line the loaf pan with baking paper.**
2. **Separate the eggs and set the egg whites to one side. Wash the lemon with hot water, dry it and rub the peel, then halve the vanilla pods and scrape out the pulp.**
3. **Mix the butter and xylitol in a large bowl to a creamy mixture. Gradually add the egg yolks.**
4. **Stir in the quark, lemon zest and vanilla pulp.**

5. Add the ground almonds and baking soda to the dough and mix well to form dough. Beat egg whites with salt until stiff and fold carefully into the dough.

6. Halve the dough and mix one half with the cocoa powder.

7. Pour the light dough into the mold and the chocolate dough on top. Mix the dough with a wooden skewer or knife to create the typical marble cake pattern.

8. Bake the cake for about 45 minutes in a preheated oven at 160 ° C (fan oven 140 ° C; gas: level 2) and let cool down a little. Serve warm or cold.

- **Vegan overnight oats with blueberries and coconut**

Nutritional values

Calories 403 kcal, Protein 15 g, Fat 22 g, Carbohydrates 35 g, Added sugar 4 g Fiber 11 g

Ingredients

- **5 tbsp oat flakes (75 g)**
- **3 tbsp coconut flakes (30 g)**
- **150 g yoghurt alternative made from soy**
- **150 ml coconut drink**
- **1 tbsp syrup (e.g. coconut blossom syrup; 15 g)**
- **100 g blueberries (fresh or frozen)**
- **2 tbsp pumpkin seeds (30 g)**

Preparation steps

1. **Mix oat flakes with 2 tbsp coconut flakes, yoghurt alternative, and coconut drink and coconut blossom syrup. Add half of the blueberries and place in the fridge for at least 2 hours, or preferably overnight.**
2. **The next morning, place vegan overnight oats with blueberries and coconut in two bowls or sealable jars. Sprinkle with pumpkin seeds and the remaining blueberries and remaining coconut flakes.**

- **Vegan overnight oats with blueberries and coconut**

Nutritional values

Calories 403 kcal, protein 15 g, fat 22 g, Carbohydrates 35 g, Added sugar 4 g Fiber 11 g

Ingredients

- **5 tbsp oat flakes (75 g)**
- **3 tbsp coconut flakes (30 g)**
- **150 g yoghurt alternative made from soy**
- **150 ml of coconut drink**
- **1 tbsp syrup (e.g. coconut blossom syrup; 15 g)**
- **100 g blueberries (fresh or frozen)**
- **2 tbsp pumpkin seeds (30 g)**

Preparation steps

1. **Mix oat flakes with 2 tbsp coconut flakes, yoghurt alternative, coconut drink and coconut blossom syrup. Add half of the blueberries and place in the fridge for at least 2 hours, or preferably overnight.**
2. **The next morning, place vegan overnight oats with blueberries and coconut in two bowls or sealable jars. Sprinkle with pumpkin seeds and the remaining blueberries and remaining coconut flakes.**

- **Keto bowl with mushrooms and Chinese cabbage**

Nutritional values

Calories 450 kcal (21%), protein 35 g (36%), fat 30 g (26%), carbohydrates 8 g (5%), added sugars 0 g (0%), Fiber 10.5 g (35%)

Ingredients

- **300 g Chinese cabbage**
- **100 g tomatoes**
- **200 g smoked tofu**
- **10 g chili pepper**
- **400 g mushrooms**
- **1 tbsp rapeseed oil**
- **salt**
- **pepper**
- **30 g macadamia nuts**
- **20 g red currants**
- **100 g soy-based skyr**
- **½ tsp medium-hot mustard**
- **1 tsp apple cider vinegar**
- **1 tbsp tahini**
- **1 stem parsley**

Preparation steps

1. Clean the cabbage, remove the outer leaves and stems, cut into fine strips, wash and drain well. Wash the tomato as well and cut into narrow strips together with the tofu. Wash, halve, core and chop the chili. Clean the mushrooms, remove the stem ends and quarter.

2. Heat the oil in a pan and fry the tofu in it over medium heat for 4–5 minutes until golden brown, then remove. Fry the mushrooms over high heat for 2-3 minutes and then remove them as well. Add cabbage, tomatoes and chili to the pan and simmer for 1–2 minutes over medium heat. Season with salt and pepper.

3. In the meantime, chop the macadamia nuts and toast them in a small pan without fat while stirring until they are fragrant. Then let it cool down.

4. For the sauce, mix the skyr, mustard, vinegar and tahini with 2 tablespoons of water and season with salt and pepper. Wash, drain and pluck currants. Wash the parsley, shake dry and also remove the leaves.

5. Divide the vegetables and tofu into bowls, add the sauce and serve sprinkled with nuts, parsley and berries.

- **Mini peppers fried in olive oil**

Nutritional values

Calories 115 kcal, Protein 1 g, Carbohydrates 4 g, Added sugars 0 g, Fiber 5 g

Ingredients

- **300 g small green pepper (preferably pimientos de padrón)**
- **2 tbsp olive oil**
- **coarse sea salt**
- **pepper**

Preparation steps

1. **Wash the peppers and dry them thoroughly with kitchen paper.**
2. **Heat the olive oil in a large non-stick pan. Add peppers and fry for 4-5 minutes over high heat, stirring constantly.**
3. **Season the paprika with coarse sea salt and pepper.**

- **Chicken and vegetable skewers**

Nutritional values

Calories 215 kcal, Protein 33 g, Fat 3 g, Carbohydrates 11 g, Added sugar 1 g,

Fiber 3 g

Ingredients

- **500 g large chicken breast fillet (2 large chicken breast fillets)**
- **3 onions**
- **2 branches rosemary**
- **2 branches thyme**
- **1 big lemon**
- **salt**
- **pepper from the mill**
- **1 tbsp olive oil**
- **700 ml kefir**
- **300 g yoghurt (1.5% fat)**
- **2 tbsp cooking cream (15% fat)**
- **1 pinch sugar**
- **2 tsp ground cumin**
- **2 fresh mint**
- **1 bunch spring onions**
- **250 g large yellow pepper (1 large yellow pepper)**
- **16 small cherry tomatoes**

Preparation steps

1. Rinse, pat dry, dice the chicken breast fillets and place in a bowl.
2. Peel the onions, dice them very finely and mix them with the poultry.
3. Wash herbs and shake dry. Strip off rosemary needles and chop finely. Also wipe off the thyme leaves. Halve and squeeze the lemon. Mix the rosemary, thyme, lemon juice and oil into the poultry cubes. Season with plenty of salt and pepper.
4. Pour the kefir over everything, mix well and cover with cling film. Let it steep (marinate) in the refrigerator for at least 5 hours, preferably overnight.
5. For the dip, stir the yoghurt with the cooking cream, sugar and cumin in a small bowl until smooth. Season to taste with salt and pepper.
6. Wash the mint, shake dry, pluck off the leaves and put some of them aside. Cut the rest into fine strips. Stir into the yogurt mixture and let it steep in the refrigerator for about 1–2 hours.
7. Clean and wash the spring onions and cut across into pieces about 2 cm long.
8. Halve, core and wash the pepper and cut into 2 cm cubes. Wash and drain the cherry tomatoes.
9. Remove the chicken cubes from the marinade and allow draining. Stick them alternately on

long kebab skewers with peppers, spring onions and tomatoes.

10. Grill on all sides for 12-15 minutes on all sides, brushing with a little marinade several times in between. Garnish the yoghurt dip with the remaining mint leaves and serve with the skewers.

- **Overnight oats with chocolate and figs**

Nutritional values

Calories 413 kcal, Protein 12 g, Fat 15 g, Carbohydrates 47 g, Added sugars 5 g,

Fiber 5 g

Ingredients

- **1-piece dark chocolate (30 g; at least 70% cocoa content)**
- **5 tbsp spelt flakes (75 g)**
- **1 tbsp cocoa powder (10 g; heavily de-oiled)**
- **200 ml oat drink (oat milk)**
- **2 tbsp pistachio nuts (30 g)**
- **2 figs**
- **2 stems mint**
- **1 tbsp cocoa nibs (10 g)**

Preparation steps

1. **Chop the chocolate and mix it with the spelled flakes, cocoa powder and oat milk and put in the refrigerator for at least 2 hours, or preferably overnight.**
2. **Roughly chop the pistachio nuts the next morning. Wash the figs, pat dry and quarter. Wash the mint, shake dry and pluck the leaves.**
3. **Put overnight oats in two bowls or sealable glasses. Spread the figs and mint leaves on**

top. Sprinkle overnight oats with chocolate and figs with chopped pistachio nuts and cocoa nibs.

- **Vegan oat porridge with mango and coconut**

Nutritional values

Calories 376 kcal, Protein 9 g, Fat 15 g, Carbohydrates 51 g, Added sugar 4 g, Fiber 8.8 g

Ingredients

- **600 ml of coconut drink**
- **200 g tender oatmeal**
- **4 tsp maple syrup**
- **400 g mango (1 mango)**
- **60 g coconut chips (6 heaped tablespoons)**
- **4 stems mint for the garnish**

Preparation steps

1. **Heat coconut drink in a saucepan. Stir in oatmeal and maple syrup and simmer for 2-3 minutes over medium heat. Then let it swell over low heat for about 5 minutes.**
2. **Meanwhile, peel the mango, cut in half and remove from the stone. Dice the pulp. Toast coconut chips in a small pan without fat over medium heat for 2 minutes. Wash mint, shake dry and pluck leaves.**
3. **Fill the porridge into glasses or bowls and garnish with mango cubes, coconut chips and mint.**

- **Buckwheat porridge with strawberries**

Nutritional values

Calories 402 kcal (19%), Protein 12 g (12%), Fat 10 g (9%), Carbohydrates 66 g, (44%), Added sugar 1 g (4%), Fiber 5.7 g (19%)

Ingredients

- **300 g buckwheat**
- **½ vanilla pod**
- **300 g strawberries**
- **400 ml oat drink (oat milk)**
- **10 g agave syrup (2 tsp)**
- **50 g almond flakes (3 tbsp)**

Preparation steps

1. **Soak buckwheat in cold water overnight. Drain the next day and rinse with clean water. Set aside 1/3 of the soaked buckwheat.**
2. **Slit the vanilla pod lengthways and scrape out the pulp.**
3. **Clean, wash and pat the strawberries dry and cut in half or into quarters depending on the size. Set aside 75 g strawberries.**
4. **Puree the oat drink with 2/3 of the buckwheat and 75 g strawberries with a hand blender. Gently heat pureed buckwheat with agave syrup and vanilla pulp in a saucepan over**

medium heat for 2 to 3 minutes, stirring regularly. Then stir in the rest of the buckwheat.

5. Fill buckwheat porridge into glasses or bowls and garnish with strawberries and flaked almonds.

- **Fish pan with Swiss chard and kohlrabi**

Nutritional values

Calories 225 kcal (11%), Protein 28 g (29%), Fat 9 g (8th%), Carbohydrates 7 g (5%), Added sugar 0 g (0%), Fiber 5.7 g (19%)

Ingredients

- **50 g onions (1 onion)**
- **1 clove of garlic**
- **600 g swiss chard**
- **300 g kohlrabi (1 kohlrabi)**
- **2 tbsp olive oil**
- **200 ml vegetable broth**
- **500 g cod fillet**
- **1 lemon**
- **100 ml cooking cream (15% fat)**
- **salt**
- **pepper**
- **1 bunch dill**

Preparation steps

1. **Peel onion and garlic and chop finely.**
2. **Wash and clean the chard. Cut out stems and dice, cut leaves into strips.**
3. **Peel and dice the kohlrabi.**
4. **Heat olive oil in a pan. Sauté the onion, garlic, chard stalks and kohlrabi cubes over a medium**

heat for 3 minutes. Pour in the broth and simmer for 5 minutes over medium heat.

5. In the meantime, rinse the fish and pat dry with kitchen paper. Halve the lemon, squeeze out and drizzle about half of it over the fish.

6. Mix the chard leaves into the cooked vegetables. Place the fish on top, pour in the cooking cream, season with salt and pepper. Cover everything and cook for about 5 minutes over medium heat.

7. In the meantime, wash the dill, shake it dry, pluck the flags from the stems and chop finely.

8. Season the fish pan with the remaining lemon juice and serve sprinkled with dill.

- **Pollack fillet with Romanesco and olives**

Nutritional values

Calories 373 kcal (18%), Protein 39 g (40%), Fat 20 g (17%), Carbohydrates 7 g (5%), Added sugars 0 g (0%), Fiber 8 g (27%)

Ingredients

- **400 g small Romanesco (1 small Romanesco)**
- **40 g green olives (without stones)**
- **2 small onions**
- **1 clove of garlic**
- **300 g pollack fillet**
- **20 g almond kernels**
- **2 stems marjoram**
- **½ lemon**
- **2 tbsp olive oil**
- **salt**
- **pepper**

Preparation steps

1. **Clean the Romanesco, cut into very small florets and wash.**
2. **Roughly chop the olives.**
3. **Peel the onions and finely dice them. Peel garlic and chop finely.**
4. **Wash the fish fillet, pat dry and cut into 3 cm pieces.**

5. Roughly chop the almonds. Wash marjoram, shake dry, pluck leaves. Squeeze the lemon.
6. Heat oil in a pan. Fry the Romanesco in it, swirling, for 3-4 minutes over high heat.
7. Add the almonds, onions and garlic and fry for 1 minute. Season with salt and pepper.
8. Season the fish pieces with pepper and add to the pan with the olives.
9. Deglaze with 2 tablespoons of lemon juice and 2 tablespoons of water. Cover immediately and cook on low heat for another 4–5 minutes. At the end of the cooking time, season with salt, sprinkle with marjoram and serve immediately.

- **Quinoa salad with spinach, grapefruit and shrimp**

Nutritional values

Calories 501 kcal (24%), protein 37 g (38%), fat 16 g (14%), carbohydrates 46 g (31%), added sugars 0 g (0%), Fiber 5.4 g (18%)

Ingredients

- **250 g quinoa**
- **625 ml vegetable broth**
- **150 g baby spinach**
- **2 grapefruit**
- **4 tbsp olive oil**
- **iodized salt with fluoride**
- **pepper**
- **600 g**
- **king prawns (12 king prawns; peeled and deveined)**

Preparation steps

1. **Rinse the quinoa under warm water until it runs clear. Cook in vegetable stock according to package instructions.**
2. **In the meantime, wash the spinach and spin dry. Fillet grapefruits, squeeze out the remaining fruit and collect the juice. For the**

vinaigrette, mix 2 tablespoons of juice with 3 tablespoons of oil, salt and pepper.

3. Rinse prawns under cold water and pat dry. Heat the rest of the oil in a pan. Fry the prawns in it over high heat for 2–3 minutes. Salt, pepper and remove from the stove.

4. Mix the quinoa with the spinach, grapefruit and prawns and drizzle with the vinaigrette.

- **Low carb zucchini pizza**

Nutritional values

Calories 678 kcal (32%), Protein 50 g (51%), Fat 47 g (41%), Carbohydrates 13 g (9%), Added sugars 0 g (0%), Fiber 4.3 g (14%)

Ingredients

- **300 g large zucchini (a 1 large zucchini)**
- **salt**
- **50 g parmesan (1 piece)**
- **1 egg**
- **125 g grated mozzarella**
- **1 clove of garlic**
- **5 tbsp tomato sauce**
- **pepper**
- **chili flakes**
- **10 g basil (0.5 bunch)**

Preparation steps

1. **Place a kitchen towel in a kitchen strainer. Wash the zucchini, grate and place in the sieve. Salt the zucchini and let it steep for about ten minutes. Then wring out the cloth with the zucchini firmly.**
2. **grate the parmesan. Mix the zucchini mass with parmesan, egg and 50 g mozzarella to a batter.**

3. Line the baking sheet with parchment paper. Put the zucchini mixture on the baking sheet and press it into a round shape, the base should be relatively thin. Bake in a preheated oven at 200 ° C (convection 180 ° C; gas: level 3) for about 20 minutes.

4. Peel and finely dice the garlic. Tomato sauce with garlic, salt, pepper and chili flakes. After 20 minutes, turn the pizza crust and spread the seasoned tomato sauce on it. Spread the rest of the mozzarella on the pizza. Bake the pizza for another 15 minutes.

5. Wash the basil, shake dry and garnish the pizza with basil leaves.

- **Rice and lentil patties**

Nutritional values

Calories 326 kcal (16%), protein 12 g (12%), fat 12 g (10%), carbohydrates 41 g (27%), added sugars 0 g (0%), Fiber 7.7 g (26%)

Ingredients

- **100 g red lenses**
- **1 aubergine**
- **1 zucchini**
- **1 yellow pepper**
- **4 tomatoes**
- **2 small onions (80 g)**
- **2 garlic cloves**
- **2 branches thyme**
- **2 branches rosemary**
- **4 tbsp olive oil**
- **iodized salt with fluoride**
- **pepper**
- **1 tsp honey**
- **1 pack reis-fit express parboiled rice**
- **100 g low-fat quark**
- **4 tbsp whole meal spelled flour (40 g)**
- **4 tbsp tender oat flakes (40 g)**
- **1 tbsp chopped parsley**
- **sweet paprika powder**

Preparation steps

1. Cook the lentils for about 15 minutes in twice the amount of water until soft, drain them and let them cool.

2. At the same time, clean and wash the eggplant, courgetti, bell pepper and tomatoes, core the bell pepper and cut everything into cubes. Peel and chop the onions and garlic. Wash herbs, shake dry and finely chop.

3. Heat 2 tablespoons of oil in a pan. Sauté the onions and garlic for 3 minutes over medium heat, remove half of the pan and set aside for the patties. Then add eggplant and zucchini cubes and fry for 5 minutes. Add the paprika and tomato cubes, season with salt, pepper, honey and herbs and cook covered for 5 minutes over low heat, stirring occasionally.

4. In the meantime, loosen the rice for the patties by gently pressing the pack, then tear open the pack. Mix rice, lentils, onion and garlic mixture that you set aside, quark, flour, oat flakes and parsley and process into a malleable mass. Season the mixture with salt, pepper and paprika powder. Shape 8 patties with your hands.

5. Heat the remaining oil in a pan and fry 4 patties on both sides for about 5–7 minutes over medium heat. Arrange patties on the ratatouille and serve.

Paella with seafood

Nutritional values

Calories 539 kcal (26%)

protein 33 g (34%)

fat 14 g (12%)

carbohydrates 69 g (46%)

added sugars 0 g (0%)

Fiber 9 g (30%)

ingredients

2 onions

2 garlic cloves

200 g cutting bean

2 red peppers

4 tbsp olive oil

250 g Oryza paella rice de valencia

400 g piece of tomato (can)

800 ml vegetable broth

2 pinch saffron threads

2 tsp hot pink paprika powder

¼ tsp dried thyme

300 g clams

250 g small squid (ready to cook)

8 king prawns (ready to cook, deveined)

salt

pepper

1 organic lemon

4 stems parsley

Preparation steps

1. **Peel and chop the onions and garlic. Clean and wash the cutting beans and cut into oblique pieces. Halve, core, wash and dice the peppers.**

2. **Heat 2 tablespoons of oil in a large pan or paella pan. Add onions and garlic and sauté for 4 minutes over medium heat. Then add rice, cutting beans and bell pepper, stir in and sauté for about 5 minutes over medium heat. Then add tomatoes and fill up with the broth. Add saffron threads, paprika powder and thyme and simmer everything for about 10 minutes over low heat. Keep stirring until the broth is almost completely absorbed.**

3. **Meanwhile, clean the mussels and wash them thoroughly under cold running water, make sure to sort out any opened mussels; these are no longer fresh. Rinse the squids, cut away any hard spots and cut the tubes into rings. Rinse the shrimp and pat dry.**

4. **Cook the mussels in boiling salted water for 8 minutes, drain and only use the opened mussels. Heat the rest of the oil in a pan, first**

fry the squids for 5 minutes over a medium heat, season with salt and pepper. Remove from the pan and fry the prawns for 5 minutes and season with salt and pepper. Spread the seafood decoratively on the paella and cover and let stand for another 5 minutes.

5. In the meantime, rinse the lemon with hot water, rub dry, cut into eighths. Wash the parsley, shake dry and pull off the leaves. Season the paella with salt and pepper and serve with lemon wedges and parsley.

- **Lentil soup with leek**

Nutritional values

Calories 289 kcal (14%), protein 11 g (11%), fat 14 g (12%), carbohydrates 29 g (19%), added sugars 0 g (0%), Fiber 6 g (20%)

Ingredients

- **150 g red lenses**
- **1 onion**
- **1 clove of garlic**
- **3 carrots**
- **1 rod leek**
- **1 red chili pepper**
- **3 tbsp olive oil**
- **15 g red curry paste (1 tbsp)**
- **30 g tomato paste (2 tbsp)**
- **100 ml apple juice**
- **750 ml vegetable broth**
- **150 ml strained tomato (glass)**
- **salt**
- **pepper**
- **½ tsp**
- **ground cumin**
- **½ tsp coriander**
- **½ tsp turmeric powder**
- **½ lemon (organic)**
- **2 spring onions**
- **2 stems parsley**

Preparation steps

1. **Rinse the lentils in a colander and let them drain. Peel onion and garlic and chop finely. Clean, peel, wash and dice the carrots. Clean and wash the leek and cut diagonally into rings. Halve the chili lengthways, remove the core, wash and chop.**

2. **Heat oil in a pot. Fry the onion, garlic, carrots and chili for 4 minutes over medium heat. Stir in the curry paste and tomato paste and sauté for 2 minutes. Then deglaze with apple juice, fill up with broth, mix in the lentils and tomatoes, stir in the spices. Let the soup simmer over low heat for 10 minutes.**

3. **Add the leek and simmer for 5 minutes, until the lentils are still bitten.**

4. **In the meantime, rinse the lemon with hot water, rub dry, rub the peel and squeeze out the juice. Clean and wash the spring onions and cut diagonally into fine rings. Wash the parsley, shake dry and chop.**

5. **Season the soup with salt, pepper and lemon juice, put in bowls, garnish with lemon zest, spring onion rings and parsley.**

- **Red apple juice with red cabbage**

Nutritional values

Calories 65 kcal (3%), protein 1 g (1%), fat 0 g (0%), carbohydrates 13 g (9%), added sugars 0 g (0%), Fiber 1.5 g (5%)

Ingredients

- **2 sweet red apples**
- **200 g red cabbage (1 piece)**
- **1 tsp balsamic vinegar**
- **ice cubes**

Preparation steps

1. **Wash, rub dry and quarter the apples.**
2. **Clean, wash and roughly chop the red cabbage. Cut a small piece into narrow strips for the garnish.**
3. **Juice the apples and red cabbage in a juicer. Mix in a glass with balsamic vinegar and ice cubes. Garnish with the red cabbage strips and enjoy immediately.**

- **Stuffed guinea fowl breast**

Nutritional values

Calories 236 kcal (11%), protein 34 g (35%), fat 6 g (5%), carbohydrates 8 g (5%), added sugars 0 g (0%), Fiber 9.5 g (32%)

Ingredients

- **1 spring onion**
- **½ tsp porcini mushroom powder**
- **250 g guinea fowl breast fillet (2 guinea fowl breast fillets)**
- **salt**
- **pepper**
- **400 g fresh sauerkraut**
- **40 g large shallots (1 large shallot)**
- **150 g beetroot (1 beetroot)**
- **2 tsp rapeseed oil**
- **4 juniper berries**
- **1 bay leaf**
- **1 pinch ground clove**
- **liquid sweetener (at will)**
- **20 g sour cream (1 tbsp)**

Preparation steps

1. **Wash and clean the spring onions, cut into fine rings and mix with the porcini mushroom powder in a small bowl.**
2. **Rinse the guinea fowl breast fillets, pat dry and cut a pocket horizontally into each one.**

3. Rub the fillets inside and outside with salt and pepper and fill with the onion and porcini mushroom mixture. Put the pockets with toothpicks.

4. Drain the sauerkraut in a colander. Peel the shallot, cut in half and cut into fine strips.

5. Wash the beetroot thoroughly, peel it and grate it roughly on a plate using a fork on a box grater or - because of the coloring beetroot juice - use rubber gloves to grate.

6. Heat 1 teaspoon oil in a saucepan or pan and fry the shallot in it until translucent. Add the grated beetroot and sauté briefly.

7. Add the drained sauerkraut, juniper berries and bay leaf and cook covered over medium heat for about 20 minutes.

8. Meanwhile, heat the rest of the rapeseed oil in a coated pan. Fry the guinea fowl fillets on both sides over medium heat for about 10-12 minutes. Season the sauerkraut with salt, pepper, cloves and, if desired, with sweetener. Serve with the guinea fowl fillets and 1 dollop of sour cream.

- **Low carb pancakes with banana**

Nutritional values

Calories 311 kcal (15%), protein 21 g (21%), fat 15 g (13%), carbohydrates 19 g (13%), added sugars 0 g (0%), Fiber 1.9 g (6%)

Ingredients

- **110 g large bananas (1 large banana)**
- **50 g almond flour (5 tbsp)**
- **2 eggs (size m)**
- **1 tsp tartar baking powder**
- **2 tsp rapeseed oil**
- **50 g blackberry**
- **100 g yogurt (3.5% fat)**
- **mint**

Preparation steps

1. **Process the banana, almond flour, eggs and baking powder in a blender or with a hand blender to a uniform mass without lumps.**
2. **Heat some oil in a pan and add 1 tablespoon of batter to each. Depending on how big you like your pancakes, the batter is enough for up to 10 (small) pancakes. Bake on both sides over medium heat for 3-4 minutes until golden brown and degrease on a kitchen towel. Wash and dry blackberries. Serve pancakes with yogurt, blackberries and garnished with mint.**

Japanese style loach fillet

Nutritional values

Calories 374 kcal (18%), protein 40 g (41%), fat 15 g (13%), carbohydrates 17 g (11%), added sugars 2 g (8%), Fiber 12.5 g (42%)

Ingredients

- **2 carrots**
- **1 yellow pepper**
- **50 g sugar snap**
- **200 g cabbage**
- **1 medium onion**
- **20 g ginger (1 piece)**
- **1 red chili pepper**
- **½ lime**
- **1 tsp sesame oil**
- **1 tbsp mirin (or dry sherry)**
- **1 tbsp soy sauce**
- **1 tsp honey**
- **320 g wolffish fillet (2 lionfish fillets)**
- **salt**
- **2 tbsp unpeeled sesame seeds**
- **2 tbsp oil**

Preparation steps

1. **Clean the carrots, bell peppers, sugar snap peas, pointed cabbage and onions, peel if necessary, wash and cut into very fine strips.**

2. Peel the ginger and cut into very fine slices. Wash the chili pepper and cut into slices (if you like it less spicy, cut it in half and remove the stones). Squeeze the lime.

3. Whisk sesame oil, 1 tbsp lime juice, mirin, soy sauce and honey with approx. 2 tbsp water to make a sauce (vinaigrette) and set aside.

4. Rinse the fish fillets, pat dry and lightly salt, sprinkle each side with sesame seeds and press down the grains a little.

5. Heat half of the oil in a non-stick pan, fry the fillets in it on the side sprinkled with sesame seeds for 1-2 minutes, turn carefully, fry for another 1-2 minutes, remove and set aside on a plate.

6. Wipe the pan with kitchen paper; add the remaining oil and heat. Fry the vegetables, chili and ginger in it over very high heat for 2 minutes while turning.

7. Place the fish on the vegetables with the sesame-sprinkled side facing up.

8. Pour in 3 tablespoons of water. Cook covered for another 4-5 minutes over medium heat, adding a little water if necessary. Arrange the vegetables and fish on plates, drizzle with the sesame and lime vinaigrette.

- **Pollack with dill potatoes**

Nutritional values

Calories 412 kcal (20%), protein 32 g (33%), fat 17 g (15%), carbohydrates 31 g (21%), added sugars 0 g (0%), Fiber 3.1 g (10%)

ingredients

- **600 g waxy potatoes e.g. b. linda**
- **2 medium onions**
- **3 tbsp rapeseed oil**
- **salt**
- **pepper from the mill**
- **200 ml vegetable broth**
- **200 ml whipped cream at least 30% fat content**
- **4 pollack fillets approx. 160 g each**
- **2 tbsp whole wheat flour**
- **½ fret dill**

Preparation steps

1. **Peel, wash, and slice the potatoes. Peel the onions, cut in half lengthways, and cut lengthways into wedges. Sauté both in 2 tablespoons of oil, season with salt and pepper, pour the broth with the cream and simmer covered for about 15 minutes.**

2. Wash pollack fillets, pat dry, season with salt, pepper, and turn in flour. Fry in the remaining hot oil for about 2-3 minutes on each side. Wash the dill, shake dry, chop, and add to the potatoes. Season the dill potatoes to taste and serve with the fish on preheated plates.

- **Fennel and pear salad**

Nutritional values

Calories 295 kcal (14%), protein 9 g (9%), fat 20 g (17%), carbohydrates 21 g (14%) added sugar 4 g (16%), Fiber 5.6 g (19%)

ingredients

- **500 g young fennel bulb**
- **120 g red seedless grapes**
- **40 g walnut kernels**
- **2 pears**
- **2 tbsp lemon juice**
- **120 g sheep cheese**
- **2 tbsp white balsamic vinegar**
- **2 tsp honey**
- **2 tbsp walnut oil**
- **jumped**
- **pepper**
- **4 stems mint**

Preparation steps

1. **Wash the fennel, cut in half, cut out the hard stalk and slice the fennel halves lengthways into thin slices. Wash, pluck, and halve the grapes. Roughly chop the nuts. Wash, peel, and quarter the pears cut out the core and cut**

the quarters into narrow wedges. Drizzle with the lemon juice.

2. Arrange the fennel with the grapes and the pears decoratively on 4 large plates. Scatter the nuts on top and crumble the feta on top. Drizzle with the vinegar, honey, and oil and season with salt and pepper.

3. Serve garnished with mint.

- **Strawberry coconut rice pudding**

Nutritional values

Calories 329 kcal (16%), protein 6 g (6%), fat 3 g (3%), carbohydrates 66 g (44%), added sugars 6.25 g (25%), Fiber 4 g (13%)

ingredients

- **1 l coconut drink**
- **I jumped**
- **250 g Oryza organic rice pudding**
- **500 g strawberries**
- **½ vanilla pod**
- **4 stems lemon balm**
- **½ bio organic lemon (zest and juice)**
- **2 tbsp agave syrup**

Preparation steps

1. **Put the coconut drink with a pinch of salt in a saucepan of at least 3 liters.**
2. **Add ORYZA organic rice pudding to the saucepan and bring to the boil. Stir occasionally. Cook the rice gently in a closed pot over low heat for 20 minutes. Stir once halfway through the cooking time. Stir well again after 20 minutes**
3. **At the same time, clean and wash the strawberries and cut lengthways into quarters.**

Halve the vanilla pod lengthways and scrape out the vanilla pulp with a knife. Wash lemon balm, shake dry, pluck the leaves, set aside some leaves for the garnish, chop the rest. Mix the strawberries with the vanilla pulp, lemon balm, grated zest and the juice of half a lemon and agave syrup.

4. Stir the rice pudding again, place in four bowls, serve with the strawberries, sprinkle with lemon balm, and serve.

- **Red mullet with a crispy crust**

Nutritional values

Calories 350 kcal (17%), protein 37 g (38%), fat 10 g (9%), carbohydrates 25 g (17%), added sugar 1 g (4%), Fiber 6 g (20%)

ingredients

- **30 g ginger (1 piece)**
- **½ lime**
- **3 tbsp soy sauce**
- **1 tbsp sweet chili sauce**
- **2 spring onions**
- **1 tbsp oil**
- **½ fret basil**
- **300 g red mullet fillet (6 red mullet fillets)**
- **salt**
- **coarsely ground pepper**
- **35 g Asian rice cookies**

Preparation steps

1. **Peel the ginger with the peeler and grate finely. Squeeze the lime and mix the lime juice with ginger, soy sauce, and chili sauce.**
2. **Clean and wash the spring onions and cut into 4 cm long pieces. Heat the oil in a pan and fry the onions over high heat for 2 minutes, stirring constantly.**

3. Deglaze with the seasoning sauce and distribute it in a baking dish.

4. Wash the basil, shake dry, pluck the leaves and pour over the onions.

5. Rinse the fish fillets, pat dry, season with salt and pepper. Place on the onion vegetable skin side up.

6. Coarsely crush Asian pastries with a spoon and sprinkle on the fish fillets. Cook in a preheated oven at 200 ° C (convection: not recommended, gas: level 3) for about 10 minutes. Lift the fish out of the mold and serve with the onion vegetables.

- **Konjac noodles with mascarpone sauce and mushrooms**

Nutritional values

Calories 582 kcal (28%), protein 12 g (12%), fat 57 g (49%), carbohydrates 5 g (3%), added sugars 0 g (0%), Fiber 5.6 g (19%)

ingredients

- **400 g mushrooms**
- **1 shallot**
- **2 tbsp olive oil**
- **400 g mascarpone**
- **100 g whipped cream**
- **1 tsp lemon juice**
- **20 g parsley (1 bunch)**
- **pepper**
- **salt**
- **nutmeg**
- **500 g konjac noodles**
- **1 small chili pepper**
- **40 g freshly grated gouda cheese**

Preparation steps

1. **Clean the mushrooms and cut them in slices. Peel and finely chop the shallot. Heat the olive**

oil in a pan and sauté the mushrooms and the shallots in it.

2. Add the mascarpone, whipped cream and lemon juice to the pan and stir, add some water if necessary and bring to the boil briefly.

3. In the meantime, wash the parsley, shake dry and chop finely. Stir half into the sauce. Season with salt, pepper, and freshly grated nutmeg.

4. Rinse konjac noodles thoroughly with water and heat in boiling salted water for 2 minutes. Then drain in a sieve, add to the sauce and mix carefully.

5. Wash and clean the chili pepper and cut into fine rings. Spread the pasta with the sauce on plates and serve sprinkled with Gouda cheese, chili, and parsley.

- **Creamy pumpkin soup with buckwheat**

Nutritional values

Calories 239 kcal (11%), protein 12 g (12%), fat 7 g (6%), carbohydrates 31 g (21%), added sugars 0 g (0%), Fiber 4.6 g (15%)

ingredients

- **200 g low-fat quark**
- **120 g buckwheat**
- **salt**
- **1 onion**
- **1 clove of garlic**
- **400 g pumpkin pulp (z. b. from pumpkin)**
- **150 g carrots**
- **2 tbsp butter**
- **400 ml vegetable broth**
- **pepper**
- **nutmeg**
- **2 stems parsley**

Preparation steps

1. **Beat the quark in a kitchen towel, screw it tightly, squeeze the quark, place the quark in a sieve, weigh it down with weights, and let it drain over a bowl.**

2. Bring the buckwheat to the boil in a saucepan with plenty of salted water and let it soak over low heat for about 30 minutes.

3. In the meantime, peel and finely chop the onion and garlic for the soup. Peel the pumpkin and carrots and cut into small cubes.

4. Melt butter in a saucepan and fry the onion with the garlic until translucent. Add diced vegetables, fry briefly, and fill up with the stock.

5. Salt, pepper, and simmer over medium heat for about 25 minutes. Puree with a hand blender and season with salt, pepper, and freshly grated nutmeg. If necessary, add a little more stock or let the soup simmer.

6. Drain the buckwheat, drain and serve with the soup. Wash the parsley, shake dry, pluck the leaves off and chop finely. Sprinkle the soup with cottage cheese and parsley and serve everything together.

- **Baked goat cheese on lettuce**

Nutritional values

Calories 291 kcal (14%), protein 10.2 g (10%), fat 26.6 g (23%), carbohydrates 3.3 g (2%), Fiber 1.3 g (4%)

ingredients

- **100 g mixed leaf salad**
- **150 g goat cheese roll**
- **50 g chopped walnut kernels**
- **50 g black olives**
- **1 tsp grainy mustard**
- **1 tsp honey**
- **2 tbsp apple cider vinegar**
- **2 tbsp olive oil**
- **salt**
- **pepper from the grinder**

Preparation steps

1. **Wash, dry, clean and cut the lettuce. Add the walnuts and olives. Cut the goat cheese into four slices and place on a baking sheet lined with baking paper. Bake under the preheated grill for about 5 minutes until golden brown.**
2. **For the dressing, stir the mustard with the honey, vinegar and oil until smooth and season with salt and pepper. Mix under the salad and**

distribute on plates. Place the warm goat cheese on top and serve.

- **Sea bass fillet the Mediterranean way**

ingredients

- **8 branches fresh thyme**
- **2 red peppers**
- **800 g ripe tomatoes**
- **1 onion**
- **2 garlic cloves**
- **300 g zucchini**
- **4 tbsp olive oil**
- **50 ml vegetable broth**
- **sea-salt**
- **pepper**
- **800 g sea bass fillet (with skin)**
- **½ lemon pressed**
- **20 g room temperature butter**

Preparation steps

1. **Wash thyme and shake dry. Halve, core, wash and dice the pepper. Wash tomatoes. For peeling, cut the tomatoes in a cross shape with a kitchen knife, scald them with boiling water for a few seconds, quench and peel them. Quarter tomatoes and cut into pieces.**

2. **Peel the onion and garlic and cut into small cubes. Wash the zucchini and thinly slice. Heat 2 tablespoons of olive oil in a pan. Add the diced vegetables and sauté for 2 minutes over**

medium heat, pour the broth on top and simmer for 2 minutes.

3. Transfer the vegetables into 4 ovenproof pans, add the zucchini slices and thyme, drizzle with the remaining oil and season with salt and pepper.

4. Wash the sea bass fillets and pat dry. Place the sea bass fillets skin up on the vegetables, brush with the butter, drizzle with a little lemon juice and sprinkle with a little salt. Bake in a preheated oven at 200 ° C (convection 180 ° C; gas: level 3) for 20–25 minutes until golden brown. Remove and serve in the pans.

- **Stewed cucumbers stuffed with minced meat**

Nutritional values

Calories 458 kcal (22%), protein 24.8 g (25%), fat 32 g (28%), carbohydrates 14.2 g (9%), added sugars 0 g (0%), Fiber 4.8 g (16%)

ingredients

- **1.6 kg braised cucumber (4 braised cucumbers)**
- **400 g ground beef**
- **300 g tomatoes (4 tomatoes)**
- **2 tbsp chopped basil**
- **1 shallot**
- **2 garlic cloves**
- **3 tbsp olive oil**
- **salt**
- **cayenne pepper**

Preparation steps

1. **Peel and finely chop shallot and garlic cloves. Sauté in hot oil, add minced meat and fry until crumbly. Remove from heat, season with salt and cayenne pepper.**
2. **Scald tomatoes with hot water, peel, quarter, core, and dice. Add to the minced meat with basil.**

3. **Peel the cucumber, cut in half lengthways, and scrape out the seeds with a spoon. Fill with minced meat, place in a casserole dish, and stew in a preheated oven at 180 ° C (convection: 160 ° C; gas: level 2–3) for approx. 15 minutes. Serve immediately.**

- **Pumpkin cream with apple**

Nutritional values

Calories 271 kcal (13%), protein 7 g (7%), fat 9 g (8%), carbohydrates 35 g (23%), added sugars 0 g (0%), Fiber 9.5 g (32%)

ingredients

- **850 g Hokkaido pumpkin**
- **1 small boskop apple**
- **1 onion**
- **2 tbsp olive oil**
- **0.7 l vegetable broth**
- **1 tsp curry powder**
- **25 g ginger in one piece**
- **4 tbsp sour cream**
- **iodized salt with fluoride**
- **pepper**
- **4 slices whole-grain bread**

Preparation steps

1. **Clean, wash, and cut the pumpkin and apple and remove the seeds. Then cut the pulp into cubes. Peel and chop the onion. Peel the ginger and grate finely.**
2. **Heat the oil in a saucepan, add the diced apple and onion and sauté for 1–2 minutes over medium heat. Add the pumpkin pulp and**

ginger and cook for 2-3 minutes. Then add the broth, bring everything to the boil, and then leave it covered over low heat for 20 minutes.

3. When the cooking time is over, add the spices and 3 tablespoons of sour cream. Puree the soup with the hand blender and season with salt and pepper.

4. Fill the ready-made soup into bowls, put a dollop of the remaining sour cream on each and serve sprinkled with pepper. Serve with whole meal bread.

- **Spring vegetable soup**

Nutritional values

Calories 71 kcal (3%), protein 5 g (5%), fat 1 g (1%), carbohydrates 11 g (7%), added sugars 0 g (0%), Fiber 7.6 g (25%)

ingredients

- **250 g red cabbage**
- **250 g white cabbage**
- **150 g celery root**
- **2 carrots**
- **250 g green asparagus**
- **1 l vegetable broth**
- **salt**
- **pepper**
- **½ fret chives**

Preparation steps

1. **Clean and wash both types of cabbage and cut into fine strips. Wash, peel and finely chop the celery and carrots. Peel the lower third of the asparagus and cut into small pieces.**

2. **Salt the broth and bring to the boil in a saucepan. Add all the vegetables and cook over low heat for about 10 minutes. Season to**

taste with salt and pepper and divide into bowls.

3. Wash the chives, shake dry, coarsely chop and serve garnished with the vegetable soup.

- **Classic vegetable soup**

Nutritional values

Calories 105 kcal (5%), protein 7 g (7%), fat 1 g (1%), carbohydrates 17 g (11%), added sugars 0 g (0%), Fiber 6.3 g (21%)

ingredients

- **150 g waxy potatoes**
- **150 g carrots**
- **150 g kohlrabi**
- **150 g green peas**
- **150 g cauliflower florets**
- **150 g celery**
- **1 ⅕ l vegetable broth**
- **salt**
- **pepper from the mill**
- **3 stems parsley**
- **2 stems lovage**

Preparation steps

1. **Peel and wash the potatoes, carrots, and kohlrabi, cut the potatoes into bite-sized pieces, roughly grate the carrots and cut the**

kohlrabi into sticks. Clean and wash the peas and cauliflower and chop the cauliflower into small pieces. Clean and wash the celery and cut it into thin slices.

2. Bring the stock to a boil in a saucepan, add the vegetables and simmer for 10–15 minutes over medium heat. Season with salt and pepper, season to taste. Wash the parsley and lovage, shake dry, chop and mix in. Divide into bowls and serve.

- **Colorful rice salad with chicken skewers and peanut dressing**

Nutritional values

Calories 613 kcal (29%), protein 42 g (43%), fat 18 g (16%), carbohydrates 70 g (47%), added sugar 1.5 g (6%), Fiber 10 g (33%)

ingredients

- **500 g chicken breast fillet**
- **10 g ginger**
- **1 clove of garlic**
- **4 tbsp sesame oil**
- **4 tbsp soy sauce**
- **250 g oryza jasmine rice**
- **salt**
- **2 carrots**
- **1 bunch spring onions**
- **200 g cabbage**
- **200 g red cabbage**
- **1 papaya**
- **1 tbsp peanut butter**
- **2 tbsp lime juice**
- **1 tsp rice syrup**
- **1 pinch cayenne pepper**
- **2 tbsp roasted peanut kernel**
- **1 handful Thai basil leaf**

Preparation steps

1. Rinse the chicken breast fillet, pat dry and cut into pieces. Put pieces on wooden skewers. Peel and finely chop the ginger and garlic. Mix 2 tablespoons of sesame oil, 2 tablespoons of soy sauce with ginger and garlic and marinate the skewers with it. Let the skewers steep in the refrigerator for about 30 minutes.

2. Put rice in a saucepan with twice the amount of cold, salted water, stir once. Then bring the water to a boil and simmer the rice in the boiling water over medium heat for 12–15 minutes. Then remove from the heat, loosen the rice and let it cool down for 10 minutes.

3. Meanwhile, clean and wash the carrots, spring onions, pointed and red cabbage and cut into fine strips. Peel papaya, cut in half, remove seeds, cut papaya into fine strips. Mix the vegetables with rice and papaya.

4. For the dressing, whisk the remaining oil, remaining soy sauce, 2 tablespoons of water with peanut butter, lime juice and rice syrup and season with cayenne pepper. Chop the peanut kernels. Wash the basil and shake dry.

5. Heat a non-stick pan and sear the skewers over medium heat on all sides for about 7-10 minutes. Arrange the salad on four plates, drizzle with the dressing, pour the skewers over it, sprinkle with the peanuts and the basil leaves.

- **Sushi bowl with salmon and avocado**

Nutritional values

Calories 526 kcal (25%), protein 21 g (21%), fat 22 g (19%), carbohydrates 59 g (39%), added sugars 5 g (20%), Fiber 6.6 g (22%)

ingredients

- **250 g oryza sushi rice**
- **5 tbsp rice vinegar**
- **2 tsp rice syrup**
- **salt**
- **4 spring onions**
- **½ cucumber**
- **200 g radish**
- **1 avocado**
- **3 stems coriander green**
- **2 tsp wasabi paste**
- **2 tbsp soy sauce**
- **2 tbsp sesame oil**
- **25 sesame seeds**
- **1 sheet nori seaweed**
- **250 g very fresh salmon fillet (sushi quality)**

Preparation steps

1. **Put the rice in a saucepan with 500 ml of water and bring everything to a boil, stirring occasionally. Let the rice cook for 2 minutes in**

an open saucepan over low heat, then cook in a closed saucepan over low heat for 15 minutes until it has completely absorbed the water. Take the pot off the stove, place a tea towel between the pot and the lid and let the rice stand for 10 minutes.

2. Meanwhile, put 3 tablespoons of rice vinegar, rice syrup and ½ teaspoon salt in a saucepan, heat and stir until the salt has dissolved. Put the sushi rice in a bowl, spread it apart so that it cools down faster. Mix in the vinegar mixture and let the rice cool down completely. Cover the sushi rice with a damp kitchen towel until further processing.

3. In the meantime, clean the spring onions, cucumber and radish, peel and wash if necessary and cut everything into very thin strips or slices. Marinate with the remaining vinegar and salt.

4. Halve the avocado, remove the stone, lift the pulp out of the skin and cut into strips. Wash the coriander, shake dry and pluck the leaves off.

5. For the dressing, mix wasabi paste with soy sauce, sesame oil, and 1 tbsp sesame seeds. Chop the nori seaweed into very thin strips. Rinse the salmon fillet, pat dry, and cut into thin slices.

6. Place the sushi rice in 4 bowls, arrange the vegetables, avocado, and salmon on top of the rice. Sprinkle with algae strips and the

remaining sesame seeds as well as coriander and serve with the dressing.

• Chicory with pomegranate seeds and bacon

Nutritional values

Calories 269 kcal (13%), protein 6 g (6%), fat 23 g (20%), carbohydrates 10 g (7%), added sugar 1 g (4%), Fiber 2 g (7%)

ingredients

- **4 chicory**
- **6 tbsp olive oil**
- **salt**
- **pepper**
- **100 g pancetta (sliced)**
- **5 g parsley**
- **½ pomegranate**
- **2 tbsp apple cider vinegar**
- **2 tsp coarse pepper**
- **1 tsp honey**

Preparation steps

1. **Clean and wash the chicory and cut in half lengthways. Heat 1 tablespoon of oil in a grill pan and grill the chicory halves on both sides for 3 minutes over medium heat. Place the**

chicory halves next to each other with the cut surface facing up in a baking dish, season with salt and pepper and bake in a preheated oven at 200 ° C (fan oven 180 ° C; gas: level 3) for 10–15 minutes

2. In the meantime, cut the pancetta into strips and fry them in a hot pan over medium heat for 4 minutes until crispy. Then drain on kitchen paper. Wash the parsley, shake dry and finely chop the leaves. Remove the pomegranate seeds from the fruit.

3. For the dressing, whisk together vinegar, mustard, salt, pepper, honey, and the remaining olive oil. Take the chicory out of the oven. Pour the dressing over the chicory halves and sprinkle with chopped parsley, pomegranate seeds, and fried pancetta.

- **Kale with raisins**

Nutritional values

Calories211 kcal (10%), protein   8 g (8 %), fat 12   g (10%), carbohydrates16 g (11%), added sugar   0   g (0%), Fiber6.4 g   (21%)

ingredients

- **400 g kale**
- **salt**
- **150 g onions**
- **1 clove of garlic**
- **2 tbsp olive oil**
- **50 g pine nuts**
- **60 g raisins**
- **2 tbsp sherry vinegar**
- **1 branch rosemary**

Preparation steps

1. **Remove the leaf veins from the kale, wash the leaves, pluck them into small pieces, shake dry and cook in boiling salted water for 3–4 minutes. Drain, quench and drain. Peel the onions and garlic, cut the onions into fine rings, chop the garlic.**
2. **Heat oil in a pan. Sauté the onion rings over a medium heat for 3 minutes while stirring. Add the garlic, raisins and pine nuts and continue**

to cook for 3 minutes while stirring. Deglaze with vinegar and simmer over low heat for about 5 minutes.

3. In the meantime, wash the rosemary, shake it dry and cut the needles into small pieces. Add the kale and rosemary to the pan and cook for another 5 minutes. Season the kale with salt and pepper,

- **Pumpkin and purple cabbage salad**

Nutritional values

Calories 405 kcal (19%), protein 13 g (13%), fat 32 g (28%), carbohydrates 16 g (11%), added sugars 0 g (0%), Fiber 8 g (27%)

ingredients

- **600 g acorn gourd (or turban gourd)**
- **140 g**
- **turkey bacon**
- **salt**
- **pepper**
- **3 tbsp olive oil**
- **600 g red cabbage**
- **3 tbsp apple cider vinegar**
- **4 tbsp walnut oil**
- **100 g physalis**
- **20 g leaf salad (e.g. red oak leaf salad, lollo rosso, radicchio, romana)**
- **30 g pumpkin seeds (2 tbsp)**
- **½ fret chives (10 g)**
- **1 tbsp lemon juice**

Preparation steps

1. **Wash, quarter and core the pumpkin and cut into 1.5 cm thick wedges. Cut the bacon into**

strips. Spread the pumpkin wedges and bacon in a baking dish, season with salt and pepper, drizzle with 1 tbsp olive oil and bake in a preheated oven at 200 ° C (fan 180 ° C; gas: level 3) for 40–45 minutes.

2. In the meantime, remove the husks and stalk from the red cabbage. Halve the cabbage, wash it, slice it into fine strips, knead with the vinegar and walnut oil, season with salt and pepper. Cover and let lettuce stand for 35–45 minutes.

3. Wash the physalis and cut in half. Wash leaf salads, spin dry and, if necessary, pluck leaves a little smaller. Toast the pumpkin seeds in a hot pan without fat over medium heat for 3 minutes. Wash the chives, shake dry and cut into fine rolls.

4. Take the mold out of the oven and let the pumpkin cool for 5 minutes. Arrange on a platter with the bacon. Spread the lettuce leaves, physalis, and red cabbage on top, sprinkle with pumpkin seeds and chives, and drizzle with the remaining olive oil and lemon juice.

- **Ginger and turmeric tea**

Material

- **1 teaspoon turmeric (10 g)**
- **2 tablespoons ginger (30 g)**
- **1 tablespoon of honey (25 g)**
- **2 cups of water (500 ml)**

How to prepare

1. **Ginger skin and grated.**
2. **Heat the water and add ginger.**
3. **Wait 5-10 minutes for it to boil.**
4. **Take the mixture out of heat and strain.**
5. **Pour the liquid into the cup and add turmeric.**
6. **Add a little honey and mix with a spoon.**
7. **Add a few drops of lemon juice to improve the taste. You can also add lemon slices if needed.**

Smoothie with pineapple and ginger

ingredients

- **1 cup fresh pineapple (150 g)**
- **1 teaspoon grated ginger (5 g)**
- **1 cup water (250 ml)**
- **1 teaspoon chia seeds (15 g)**

Method of preparation

1. **Mix all ingredients in a blender or juicer.**
2. **Process them at high speed until you get a fine texture.**
3. **Pour the smoothie into a glass and drink it immediately to assimilate all the nutrients.**

- **Smoothie with Pineapple and Celery**

ingredients:

- **2 cups (400 ml) of water**
- **2 cups (300 g) of fresh pineapple**
- **1 stalk of celery**
- **The juice obtained from half a lemon**
- **1 tablespoon (25 g) of honey**

Method of preparation:

1. **The ingredients presented above are enough to prepare two glasses of smoothie with pineapple and celery. The first glass should be consumed on an empty stomach in the morning and the second at noon.**
2. **Try to buy organic pineapple and celery. This is the only way to be sure that these two ingredients offer you maximum benefits.**
3. **The first step is to slice the pineapple until you manage to fill two cups, then wash and slice the celery. Squeeze the juice of half a lemon and you're done with the first phase.**
4. **The second step involves putting all the mentioned ingredients (the two cups of water, pineapple, celery, lemon juice and a spoonful of honey) into a food processor. Process for a few seconds until you get a homogeneous liquid.**

Green Tea With Pineapple And Cinnamon?

ingredients

- **A cup of water (250 ml)**
- **½ teaspoon ground cinnamon (2 g)**
- **A teaspoon of green tea (5 g)**
- **2 slices of pineapple**
- **2 teaspoons honey (50 g)**

Method of preparation

1. **Bring the water to a boil and add the ground cinnamon.**
2. **Boil water for at least 2 minutes. Then add the green tea.**
3. **Meanwhile, extract the juice from the pineapple slices.**
4. **After boiling the tea, let it cool to room temperature for 8-10 minutes.**
5. **When the infusion is lukewarm, add pineapple juice and honey.**
6. **Mix well and consume while still warm.**

- **Sharp carrot juice with curry foam**

ingredients

- **½ small lime**
- **1 stem coriander**
- **½ tsp mild curry powder**
- **½ tsp hot curry powder**
- **150 ml carrot juice**
- **30 ml milk (1.5%; preferably long-life milk)**

Preparation steps

1. **Squeeze half a lime.**
2. **Wash the coriander, shake dry, pluck the leaves and cut into fine strips.**
3. **Mix the mild and hot curry powder in a small bowl.**
4. **Put the carrot juice and lime juice with 2/3 of the curry mixture in a tall container and mix briefly with a hand blender.**
5. **Mix the rest of the curry mixture with the milk and use a milk frother to create a fine-pored, stiff foam. Put the carrot juice in a tall glass, place the curry foam on top with a spoon, sprinkle with coriander and enjoy.**

Tomato and Apricot Fresher

ingredients

- **600 ml tomato juice**
- **2 bay leaves**
- **salt**
- **pepper**
- **cayenne pepper**
- **1 lemon**
- **4 stems basil**
- **4 apricots**
- **350 ml cold sparkling mineral water**
- **ice cubes**

Preparation steps

1. **Heat the tomato juice with bay leaves, a little salt, pepper, and cayenne pepper in a saucepan. Squeeze the lemon, add the juice to the tomato juice, bring to the boil, and boil for 5 minutes over medium heat. Remove from heat, let cool down a bit and then place in the fridge for 1 hour.**

2. **In the meantime, wash the basil, shake dry and pluck the leaves. Put 4 leaves aside, cut the rest into fine strips. Wash apricots, rub dry, cut in half and remove the stones. Cut the apricot halves into thin slices.**

3. **Remove bay leaves from tomato juice; Finely puree half of the apricots with the juice and spread over 4 glasses with basil strips. Top up with sparkling water and ice cubes, add apricot wedges and garnish with basil leaves. Serve immediately.**

• **Avocado chocolate mousse**

ingredients

- **2 ripe avocados**
- **2 tbsp coconut milk**
- **40 g cocoa powder**
- **40 ml of honey**
- **½ tsp vanilla powder**
- **½ tsp chia seeds (ground)**
- **12 raspberries**
- **1 tsp grated coconut**

Preparation steps

1. **Halve the avocados, stone them and spoon them into a blender.**
2. **Add coconut milk, cocoa powder, honey, vanilla powder and ground chia seeds.**
3. **Puree to a creamy mass.**
4. **Chill at least 30 minutes or overnight before serving. Pick out the raspberries, wash, and pat dry. Garnish the avocado and chocolate mousse with raspberries and coconut flakes.**

- **Avocado mint ice cream with chocolate**

ingredients

- **400 ml coconut milk (can)**
- **3 ripe avocados**
- **10 g mint (0.5 bunch)**
- **2 tbsp lemon juice**

- **50 g agave syrup**
- **100 g chocolate drops made from dark chocolate (cocoa content at least 70%)**

Preparation steps

1. **Open the coconut milk and spoon out the solid part at the top - do not shake the can beforehand - and place it in a large bowl. Whisk the firm coconut milk with a hand mixer and then pour it into a cake or baking dish.**
2. **Halve the avocados, remove the stones, remove the pulp, and put in a blender. Wash mint, shake dry, and pluck leaves. Puree the avocado pulp with lemon juice, agave syrup, and mint to a creamy and smooth mass.**
3. **Pour the avocado mixture onto the frothy coconut cream, sprinkle with chocolate drops and mix the mixture carefully but evenly. The surface of the mass should be relatively smooth.**
4. **Place cling film on the ice cream mass and press down lightly so that there is no air between the film and the ice cream mass. Place the ice in the freezer for at least 2 hours.**

Let it thaw briefly and enjoy.

- **Pineapple popsicles**

ingredients

- **600 g fresh pineapple pulp**
- **100 g raspberries**

- **200 g coconut cream (without sugar)**
- **50 g rice syrup**
- **1 lime (juice)**

Preparation steps

1. **Cut the pineapple pulp into pieces, put 100 g aside. Wash the raspberries carefully and pat them dry.**
2. **Mix coconut cream with rice syrup. Put the pineapple together with the coconut cream and the lime juice in a blender and mash finely.**
3. **Fill the mixture into 8 ice cream molds, add 4-5 raspberries each and let freeze for about 1 hour. Then insert wooden sticks and let it freeze for another 3 hours. To serve, remove ice from the molds and arrange with the pineapple pieces set aside.**

- **Coconut and chocolate ice cream with chia seeds**

ingredients

- **400 ml of coconut milk**
- **4 tbsp maple syrup**

- **15 g cocoa powder (2 tbsp; heavily oiled)**
- **2 bags chai tea**
- **12 g white chia seeds (2 tbsp)**
- **250 g soy yogurt**
- **30 g dark chocolate (at least 70% cocoa)**

Preparation steps

1. **Put coconut milk in a saucepan. Add maple syrup and cocoa powder and heat, but do not bring to the boil. Hang the tea bag in, cover, remove from the heat, and let steep for 30 minutes. Then take out the tea bag, squeezing out the liquid. Mix in 1 1/2 tbsp chia seeds and yogurt.**
2. **Fill the mass in 8 ice molds and let freeze for about 1 hour. Then insert wooden sticks and let them freeze for another 3 hours.**
3. **Chop the chocolate and melt over a warm water bath. Remove the ice cream from the molds and decorate with the chocolate and the remaining chia seeds.**

CONCLUSION

Weight loss is a huge problem that most people face early in their lives. May it be a struggle or need to do to maintain a healthier body and lifestyle, consuming nutritious foods to lose weight makes the job easier. To minimize calorie intake, count your every bite. It is to assess the amount of calories you need to develop your muscle and provide the body with adequate nutrients as well as slashing those pounds.

When trying to lose weight, eating nutritious foods will go along with taking up as many nutrients as possible, while reducing calorie intake as normal. This balance must be known, because most people underestimated this method and end up eating poorly. This is a very bad strategy because eating poorly when decreasing weight can result in muscle loss along with fat, which can also lead to energy loss.

Clean fruits and vegetables are the great foods to lose weight. Also, strawberries, citrus fruits and vegetables such as green peppers and tomatoes make a perfect addition because they are low in calories and contain vitamin C. The form of food to include is avocadoes. This fiber-high fruits have omega-3 fatty acids that are not only healthy for the skin, but also play a very important role in brain function and in our normal growth and development.

The amount of food consumption is essential to healthy eating and weight loss. However if these are foods to lose weight, the intake should also be regulated. Low-fat meats and even balanced fish such as salmon should be consumed in minimum amount, a deck card size would do. A cup of fresh steamed green beans or broccoli provides a nutritious addition with a single slice of whole grain bread.

In order to understand why diet is so important in weight loss, we need to remember something key. Our body is nourished by the food we eat. In other words, food is our source of energy, something like our "essence". We must, therefore, promote the consumption of healthy and nutritious food so that all food is used as a source of energy. When we eat excessively fatty foods, what we are doing is storing that fat in our body. The point is that our body can hardly take advantage of this fat, so it is stored in the body as a reserve source of energy.